FOR GIVING
LOVE

Awakening Your Essential Nature
Through Love and Forgiveness

LEONARD LASKOW, M.D.
WITH
STEVE BHAERMAN

To Sama, my dear wife.
Without her this book would not have been written.

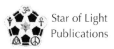 Star of Light
Publications

Publisher: Jesse Krieger

Write to Jesse@JesseKrieger.com if you are interested in publishing through Star
of Light Publications or foreign rights acquisitions of our catalogue books.

Learn More: www.JesseKrieger.com

TABLE OF CONTENTS

PREFACE

When I set out to write *For Giving Love*, I realized that most of the great works of art are created not with the audience in mind but as a creative expression of the Divine — an expression that simply must be manifested. You didn't arrive here to live your life for others, or to express what others think, value and want. You're living your life because life lives itself through you. Yes, you can choose to take this life force and devote it to the well-being of others, but the life force didn't come here for that; it came here to just express itself. In other words, life is to be lived and has an inherent impulse to become conscious of itself. And Essence is simply a sense of being. To be aware of being, and then to share it as part of the complexity called awakening is what *For Giving Love* is really about.

Leonard Laskow, M.D. December 2015

INTRODUCTION:

ON LOVE
AND FORGIVENESS

And the day came when the risk to remain tight in a bud was more
painful than the risk it took to blossom.
— Anaïs Nin

It is not how much we give but how much love we put into giving.
— Mother Teresa

Love is the unconditional acceptance of what is.
Leonard Laskow

If you're holding this book in your hands — or reading it on
your screen — you already have some curiosity about forgiveness.
Perhaps you've had a profound experience of forgiveness yourself
or seen how it has transformed the life of another. Or maybe you're
skeptical about forgiveness because you imagine that it's a way of
pretending to make something all right when it isn't or condoning

something that cannot be condoned.

It is my hope that this book will transform your experience of forgiveness and give you lifelong tools for generating genuine peace and healing in your life and in the world. You may be surprised to discover that your assumptions about what forgiveness is have been limited by misinformation or missing information. You may be relieved to find that forgiving has nothing to do with forgetting, denying, or condoning horrors. It is not about anyone else "out there."

It is about how YOU are holding the circumstance. When you release identification with or an attachment to the past then…

Forgiving is for giving love…
and for giving freedom.

Forgiving is a way of clearing the spiritual "palate" for the next taste of life and for truly loving yourself more deeply — or perhaps for the first time. Forgiving frees you from the past and frees you to be who you really are. With the energy of the past cleared, we are free from the emotional charge of old stories, conditions, and patterns … and free to be fully present.

This book will offer you a clear and practical pathway for forgiving. It will offer inspiring stories of those who have transformed their lives through the Holoenergetic Forgiveness Process. You'll learn how forgiving changes you on a cellular level — the biology of forgiveness — and how it can change the field around you so that other people you haven't spoken with in years suddenly have a change of heart.

You'll learn about what I call "the Game of Awakening," an operational cosmology that will give you otherworldly resources to deal with this-worldly challenges. I've found that this operational cosmology helps seminar participants negotiate the unmanifest that is beyond the understanding of the thinking mind.

You'll also learn what forgiveness is and is not, and perhaps gain some insight into why forgiveness may have been challenging for you until now — and why it can lead to the next level of breakthrough in your life. You will learn how to practice "presence" so you can look at any situation through the eyes of your soul. Of course you will learn the Holoenergetic Forgiveness Process and be inspired by stories of how forgiveness heals. And you will get a glimpse of what is "beyond" forgiveness — a world where presence is being alive and aware here and now.

Whatever condition or situation you find most challenging in life — whether that be health, relationships, money, career, or overall happiness — forgiveness has the power to release the blocks that have been keeping you from unconditionally loving yourself exactly as you are.

Forgiveness has the power to release the blocks that have been keeping you from unconditionally loving yourself exactly as you are

---

At this point you might also be wondering how someone trained as a scientist, and as a medical doctor, could get so involved with healing through love and forgiveness.

So … a bit of background.

What brought me to the realizations I share with you in these pages began in the 1970s with my discovery of the healing effects of love, which was documented in my first book, Healing with Love: A Breakthrough Mind/Body Medical Program for Healing Yourself and Others. At the time of its publication, Deepak Chopra said my work revealed that "Love is truth and beyond sentiment …the ultimate healer." Since then, my research, healing work, further discovery, and teaching have continued. I present it here in a rich, practical way that can be applied to every area of our lives, and most certainly for our own inner development and for a deepening realization of our essential wholeness.

Healing with Love

My immersion in forgiveness and healing with love began at a retreat in the mid-1970s. It was about 2:00 a.m. and I was in deep meditation, alone in my dark room. Suddenly it felt like someone had turned on the lights. I opened my eyes and the room was still dark. I closed my eyes, and again I experienced this inner luminosity. I then felt a presence and heard a voice inside my head. I say it was a voice, but it was indescribable, not audible in the usual sense. This presence said, "Your work is to heal with love." The hair stood up on the back of my neck and tears started to roll down my cheeks. I knew what was said was true but I didn't know what it meant.

Then I silently said, "Oh, so I'm worthy!"

In response, this voice, this presence, said, "You are no more or less worthy than anyone else. Your work is to heal with love."

In other words, when the conditioned, egoic sense of the self that we sometimes call the little self asked, "Am I really good enough?" this presence would have nothing to do with the judgment or comparison that "worthy" implied. I took this information in, although at that stage in my life I really had no idea what to do with it. At the time, I was in a busy medical practice in San Francisco and teaching at the University of California San Francisco Medical Center.

For years, I couldn't speak about this experience. It had been so profound, so ineffable.

Less than a year later, I was at another retreat. My roommate was a young man in his early thirties. He was from Australia and a composer of children's songs. As it turned out he had metastatic cancer. He had ten golfball-sized lesions in one lung and seven in another. One of his kidneys was completely obstructed with cancer. The other one was fifty percent functional.

In the middle of the first night, I was awakened by my roommate crying out in pain. He was having trouble breathing, so I got up, went over to his bed and asked, "Can I help?"

"Anything, mate," he said.

I had no medication handy, so I just sat down on his bed and visualized above my head a radiant sphere of light like the sun with a beam of light descending through the top of my head to the center of my chest. From there the energy flowed out from my heart, up my shoulders, and down my arms. I held my hands on both sides of his chest, recreated this radiant sun between my hands, and just held it there without any particular thought or intention. This all occurred spontaneously, without my stopping to think about what I was doing or why.

Almost immediately he began to breathe more easily and in a few moments he said, "Thanks, Doc. The pain is gone. The pain is gone."

He slept well for the rest of that night. The next morning when he woke up, he said, "Hey, Doc, you know, you're really a healer."

Healing with love, I thought. What had happened that night? I didn't know. I only knew that it had been something very profound, beyond my understanding at the time.

Now if I were to go to a standard Textbook of Medicine and look up the word "love," or "healing with love," I would find nothing about it there. Interesting, considering that love is the oldest and the most powerful force for healing that humanity has ever known, yet it had never been acknowledged or explored by the medical profession.

Love is the oldest and the most powerful force for healing that humanity has ever known, yet it had never been acknowledged or explored by the medical profession.

This is what prompted me to start my own exploration of love and healing.

For the next few days my roommate had no more pain and slept well. And then, following the retreat, we hugged and said good-bye.

He was returning to Peter Bent Brigham Hospital at Harvard to receive chemotherapy. While receiving chemotherapy, he had an epiphany that he was being guided by Source, and that all was well. Several days later, X-rays revealed that the lung and kidney tumors were no longer present. He had what is called a "spontaneous remission," meaning conventional medicine was unable to explain how the tumors resolved.

About ten years later, at another conference, I heard a man singing children's songs and he started to tell his story about his illness and his healing. Could it be? Yes, it was the man I'd met at the retreat. I went up to him and asked, "Do you remember me?"

"Of course," he said. "Doc, you pulled me through when I was going under."

We hugged and there were tears. As I thought about what had occurred, I knew that I personally had nothing to do with his healing because I literally didn't do anything. I was a conduit for whatever portion of this gift of grace I was to be part of. But that early experience of healing and love started a long process of exploration for me that continues to this day.

When I returned to my medical practice, I started looking for opportunities to explore what I had experienced. As a medical practitioner, a guiding principle was to knowingly do no harm either by commission or omission. We all know the classical medical invocation, "First, do no harm." At the same time, if I had a sense that something could be helpful — even if it was beyond my or the patient's understanding — I felt inclined to try it.

One day, a patient came in who had a pelvic mass. It was actually an old pelvic inflammatory disease process. In the past she had had an infection in her fallopian tube, which had filled with pus. It had been treated with antibiotics and was no longer active. She had just gotten married and had found intercourse with her husband painful, and this was affecting their relationship. When I examined her, I felt this mass, which was about six centimeters in diameter with some tenderness associated with adhesions to the side wall of the pelvis.

"What can we do?" she asked.

The mass was large enough to warrant surgery, which I offered her.

Then she asked, "Is there anything else?"

Since she didn't have an active infection, antibiotics would be of no value. The symptoms were caused by the adhesions from the previous infection and I knew that a delay of a week before doing surgery would do no harm. So I answered, "Well, we could do energy work."

"What's that?" she asked.

I didn't know quite how to answer, how to describe what it was. "Well," I said. "Let's just do it."

"Uh…okay," she said.

I did the same thing that I had done with the young man with metastatic cancer. I sensed and imagined a radiant sun between my hands and held it like that for three or four minutes. When I felt a sense of completion I said, "Well, we're done."

"Is that it?"

"Yes, come back in a week for a follow up."

A week went by and she didn't return. And I thought, uh-oh, maybe I'd made a big mistake. What if the Board of Medical Examiners asked what I had done to treat this person?

Anyway, I decided I couldn't continue to explore this healing work in the context of my medical practice, so I stopped thinking about it. Nine months later I saw my patient's name on my appointment calendar, the same woman for whom I'd done the healing work. And it's interesting that it was nine months later because I'm an obstetrician-gynecologist. Nine months. She came in and I asked her how she was feeling.

"Fine," she said. "Everything's fine."

I did a follow-up exam. There was no mass, no induration (hardness), and no tenderness. I asked her why she hadn't returned in a week as we'd scheduled.

"After you treated me," she replied, "I had no more problems. So I thought, why come back?"

This encouraged me to do similar work with select patients, and with gynecologic issues as well as infertility, hypertension and rheumatoid arthritis. While I was getting excellent results, I still didn't understand the real nature of these healing processes but felt it was important to explore them.

Clearly what I was doing worked, although I didn't know why. As a physician trained in the scientific tradition, I had to consider that at least in part the results were due to the placebo effect. I knew, of course, that if you give somebody a sugar pill and tell them that it's a medication, approximately thirty percent of patients get the healing effect they've been told it will produce. Some people even grow hair when they're told a certain medication grows hair. That's the power of belief. However, I was quite certain there was something more than the power of belief associated with what I'd witnessed in the healing work with patients. So I decided to explore this in a disciplined and systematic way.

I wondered how much of what I'd witnessed with my patients had been a manifestation of the body-mind response currently being explored in the field of epigenetics. ("Epi" means above, so epigenetics refers to something beyond the genes, something in the environment having an impact on genetic expression.) As Albert Einstein said, "The field is the sole governing force over the particle." The particles of matter that comprise the human body are subject to an invisible field that moves the particles around, similar to the way a magnet moves iron filings. Could the interaction between my consciousness and the consciousness of the person I was working with have such an impact on the physical body? I was determined to find out.

The particles of matter that comprise the human body are subject to an invisible field that moves the particles around, similar to the way a magnet moves iron filings.

Through the subsequent study of epigenetics, we now know that perceptions, beliefs, interpretations, and judgments (for example, the belief, "I'm not good enough") can lead to a sense of separation, which in turn has physiological ramifications. The stress, fear, anxiety, anger, and depression brought on by these feelings of separation stimulate the release of cortisol and adrenaline. These hormones, when chronically released as a response to "normal life" — as opposed to imminent danger — can cause degenerative illnesses such as hypertension, cancer, heart disease, autoimmune disease, and diabetes.

All these perceptions, beliefs, interpretations, and judgments veil us from our essential nature. Fortunately, there are processes outlined in this book — the Tracing, Forgiveness and Unconditional Love processes — that dissolve these veils of separation and reconnect us with our essential nature. These stimulate the positive epigenetic signals of unity, love, joy, happiness and peace — feelings that release the feel-good hormones and neurotransmitters like oxytocin, dopamine, prolactin, atrial natriuretic peptide and endorphins.

At the time I conducted my experiments, epigenetics was in its infancy, and we didn't know the full effect of the environment on our genetic predisposition. It has since been said that "genetics loads the gun, but environment pulls the trigger."

We did know about the placebo effect, the phenomenon I referred to earlier, where just the belief that one is being healed has positive physiological consequences. To rule out the placebo effect, I decided to focus my research on single-celled organisms such as bacteria, tumor cells, and also on water and DNA, which as far as we know don't have beliefs.

For the next phase of my investigation, I collaborated with a friend of mine, Dr. Glen Rein, a neurobiologist who was working at a major university in the San Francisco Bay area. What I soon discovered would reveal a whole new level of understanding, not only of the healing process but also the power and nature of love.

An Epiphany on Unconditional Acceptance

Since major universities rarely have financial endowments for "healing with love," I had to conduct my research "after hours" when the laboratories were available. My first pilot research project was with salmonella, a bacterium that causes dysentery in humans. And in preparation for beginning my work, I was looking at the bacteria under a microscope and had a deep realization — an epiphany. It suddenly struck me that the same Source that created me, created these bacteria. And these bacteria had as much right to exist as I did.

It suddenly struck me that the same Source that created me, created these bacteria. And that these bacteria had as much right to exist as I did.

——

In that moment all the conditioned filters in consciousness from my medical training dissolved.

I felt a transcendent connection with All of Life — including the salmonella. And there was only this consciousness and the consciousness of the bacteria, vibrating at the same frequency, because at the transcendent level of consciousness, all is One.

Subsequently, while recreating this field of Oneness and connectedness, if I introduced the intention for the bacteria to reduce its growth rate ... it did so by fifty percent compared to controls as measured by an optical density spectrophotometer.

Just as years earlier, when I had been awed by the message about healing with love, and just as I had seen that mysterious power manifest with me as the conduit, I now had another key piece related to love. In the space of unconditional loving acceptance and Oneness,

I was able to influence the growth of "harmful" bacteria by linking with its consciousness and introducing the intention to change its behavior. In other words, instead of seeking to kill the bacteria, I acknowledged its right to live and simply intended to change its behavior (i.e., growth rate).

When I unconditionally accepted its right to exist, I entered into a state of Oneness with the consciousness of the bacteria, and from that state of Oneness, I was able to influence its behavior.

At that point, I had another realization. This unconditional acceptance of "what is" is another way of talking about unconditional love. Just stop for a moment and consider what it would be like if you were unconditionally accepted, right here, right now, exactly as you are. What would you feel? You would feel unconditionally loved. Then the question arose in me. If you unconditionally love this bacteria, why are you wanting to change it? Well, I reasoned, you are changing its behavior, not its right to exist. You can, for example, unconditionally love your child. What if this young child were behaving wildly and running across a busy intersection? You could unconditionally love your child, AND want to change its behavior.

The entire idea of "intervention" in the area of addiction was developed as an expression of unconditional love and acceptance — AND — wanting to change someone's behavior as an expression of that love. Loved ones can do interventions because they love someone unconditionally and are taking a stand to support that individual's Being beyond the addictive condition.

The practices and processes introduced in this book — like the Aware Witness Practice and the Holoenergetic Forgiveness Process — are designed to help you do an intervention on yourself, so that you can love yourself without condition. In doing that fundamental healing, you may see many "conditions" clearing up spontaneously.

Speaking of unconditional love, we extended that love to the bacteria as well in a novel way. We wondered if this loving energy could protect bacteria from the lethal effects of antibiotics. We did a series of elegant, well-controlled experiments that indicated that love could protect bacteria from the lethal effects of antibiotics, if we so intended. The purpose of the experiment was to explore the power of love beyond the placebo effect.

I then began to work with cancer cells grown in tissue culture. I tried five different thought intentions and found the most powerful one to be, "Return to the natural order, harmony, structure, and function of your pre-hyperactive cell line."

Since cancer cells grow at an accelerated rate, this intention — again, in a field of loving acceptance — slowed their rate of growth. The experiment involved three different expressions of intention: thought, imagery, and thought and imagery combined. When we used just the thought intention, we got a twenty-percent reduction in the growth rate of cancer cells grown in tissue culture. When we used imagery, we also got a twenty-percent reduction. However, when we added thought and imagery together, we got a forty-percent reduction. Our conclusion was that for the best results, when creating an intention, use both thought and imagery.

It was through this work that I was convinced beyond my own skepticism that love is not just the stuff of mystics and poets and romantic movies. It is the universal harmonic that has the power to influence the material world, making it the most powerful subtle energy we know of.

Love is the universal harmonic that, through the resonance of relatedness, brings us into unity.

You can read about these experiments in greater detail in my book, Healing with Love and in the article, "Healer Intention," in the appendix of this book.

This book is designed to pick up where that one left off and address more specifically how YOU can bring the very tangible power of love and forgiveness into your world. You will learn why forgiveness works, not just in metaphysical terms, but also biologically. You will come to recognize the patterns and beliefs that create resistance to forgiveness, and you will see clearly how easy it is to overcome this resistance once you understand what a powerful force forgiveness is. You will learn how to practice "presence" so that who you really are can compassionately transcend who you "think" you are. And, you will learn a simple, easy-to-use process to help you forgive and free yourself from past limitations and stories to finally be who you really are.

You will also have the opportunity to unconditionally love and accept yourself — and in so doing, become a light unto the world.

Thank you in advance for joining me on this transformational journey, and may the power of Love light your way.

FOR GIVING
LOVE

CHAPTER 1

THE GAME
OF AWAKENING

Realize deeply that the present moment is all you ever have.
Make the Now the primary focus of your life.
— Eckhart Tolle

Love is an awakening to Oneness at the deepest level, an acknowledg-
ment of the unity of every thing.
— Leonard Laskow

While this is a book on forgiveness, forgiveness is part of a much
larger context that I call the Game of Awakening. What do I mean
by that? Why "awakening"?

There is the classic story of the Brahman priest asking Buddha
if he was a divine being — a god or demi-god — and Buddha's response was, "I am awakened."

Awakened to what?

The traditions would suggest Buddha — and others who have

experienced a deep and profound epiphany of life beyond this veil — awakened to the illusory nature of what we call reality, recognizing that we are not just our physical bodies, our thoughts, beliefs, sensations, emotions and the material conditions and "stuff" that manifest in our lives.

Buddha awakened to recognize both the form and the formless, the manifest and the unmanifest as the One. You may be thinking, "I picked up this book because I am seeking to make this life better — greater happiness, improved health, better relationships, greater satisfaction from my work. Are you saying that all of this is an illusion?"

Not exactly.

You will see as you read on, by playing the Game of Awakening, we release our attachment to outcome. Out of this freedom we may spontaneously manifest those things we desire — because we don't HAVE TO have them to be happy.

Interestingly, once we realize our happiness is a place we are coming from, not going to, our specific desires for certain things or conditions become preferences rather than addictions. From the standpoint of this deeper awakening, we recognize that desires, like thoughts and feelings, are waves that arise and subside in the ocean of awareness, impermanent forms returning to the formless realm from which they arose. In this way, transcendent awareness of who we really are releases attachment to form and outcome — and we are happy just to Be.

Happiness is a place we are coming from, not going to.

Awakening can happen in stages, and it can happen all at once. As you read in the introduction, I had a spiritual revelation that my mission was to heal with love. I was fortunate to experience how love heals physical conditions in humans — as well as how it can influence the growth of bacteria, cancer cells, and DNA.

It wasn't until several years later that I had an experience where I pierced the veils in my own life.

A Near-Death Experience

In the early 1980s, a friend of mine who was Chief of Orthopedic Surgery at Marin General Hospital, near my home just north of San Francisco, had given me $10,000 worth of surgical instruments as a gift to deliver to a hospital in Bali. He also introduced me to the American Vice Consul in Bali, who told me a story that piqued my curiosity. She was married to a Balinese at an outdoor wedding on a day when it was raining heavily. One of the wedding guests was her husband's uncle, who said, "Don't worry about the weather. I'll take care of it."

Apparently, the uncle was a shaman. He went into a room, and before long it stopped raining around the house. People arriving from all directions said it was raining everywhere — except in the courtyard where the wedding was taking place. For three hours, there was no rain. Then, when the ceremony was over, it began raining again.

Intrigued, I told her I would like to meet this "uncle," who lived up in the mountains and had no telephone. A few days later, we drove up to the village to meet him. He was in his mid-fifties at the time, thin of stature, and nearly toothless. I told him I was interested in learning how he did this, and he said through an interpreter, "If you're really interested, you'll have to come back and stay with me for three months."

When my host mentioned that I was from California and facilitated healing from the heart, he said — again through an interpreter — "Let's see if you can penetrate my energy field with your energy."

I was reluctant to engage in whatever kind of shamanic competition he had in mind, but he insisted that I try it. He held his breath and established a strong energy field, and I half-heartedly held up my hand. He seemed happy that it appeared I was unable to penetrate his energy field. He then told me he had a problem with his heart and asked if I would do some healing work with him. So I aligned with him, heart to heart. Little did I realize that he was using this opportunity to drain MY energy!

I aligned with the shaman, heart to heart. Little did I realize that he was using this opportunity to drain MY energy!

When I was done working with him, he brought over what looked like a small set of venetian blinds with images and symbols. He said, "Here is how I do my work. If I focus on this image here, I send energy to people and they feel good. When I focus on this energy on the left, they feel bad."

I asked him who decides whether good energy or bad energy is sent. "I do," was his reply. This didn't raise a red flag for me, probably because I'm from California, the land of love, light, and naiveté. I had not been exposed to Balinese black-and-white magic shamanism before.

We drove down from the mountain, and later that day I was at the Café Lotus to do some healing work on the cafe manager. As the sun began to set, I started to feel some pain in my heart. I flashed on an old Australian saying, "Never get sick in Bali." Apparently, there are all sorts of stories about folks waking up in the hospital after an accident minus a limb. This is the reason I was bringing the gift of surgical instruments.

I had rented a hut in a rice paddy for the night, and the manager and I walked half a mile to get there. As I did healing work with him, my energy grew weaker and weaker. Afterward, I felt exhausted and more pain in my heart. By the time darkness had set in, there was no position I could remain in without feeling intense pain —

and weakness. I gave my girlfriend my passport with the expectation I would need to be evacuated — and with the sense I was unlikely to make it through the night.

Later in the night an incident occurred. There was a fly buzzing around me and bothering me. At one point I snatched the fly out of the air in the complete darkness. Was this the shaman, shifting shape to "bug" me and further drain my energy? I knew that without divine intervention, there was no way I could have reached out in the dark and caught the fly by myself. In that moment, I felt Source was with me and I would make it through the night.

The pain stopped at dawn. I was able to walk from the hut on my own, went to the hospital and got a cardiogram. The doctor diagnosed it as "coronary insufficiency" and prescribed rest and medication. So I went to a hotel on the beach, thinking that if I were to transition, I'd rather do it in a tropical setting with a magnificent view.

I went to bed, my girlfriend went into town, and once again, as the sun began to set, the pain set in. This time I KNEW I wouldn't last the night. I meditated and said goodbye to my loved ones, and knowing there was nothing else that could be done, I surrendered to Source. I released all intention and effort, and found myself moving down a dark tunnel toward an extraordinary light, where I saw this radiant light Being, and a crowd of Beings behind it.

Then suddenly, BOOM! I was back. The pain was completely gone and I was at peace. I knew beyond understanding that I had experienced Ever-present Home, and from that moment I have had no fear of death.

I knew beyond understanding that I had experienced Ever-present Home, and from that moment I have had no fear of death.

The next morning, I received a call from the cafe manager, whom I'd done healing work on two days before. He told me the Vice Consul was arranging to evacuate me to the American Hospital in Singapore. Apparently he had heard of my experience with "uncle" because he asked me, "Do you know who you were dealing with? You were with the master black magician of Bali who meditates every night in the Temple of Death."

Uncle, the man told me, would have battles with other magicians on the beach. They would throw "energy" and try to kill one another. If he could extract more energy from someone — particularly someone he perceived to have healing energy, like me — he would do it to gain advantage. Nothing personal. Just as you or I might be hungry for food, his "unholy hunger" was for life energy. He perceived me to be weaker than he was but strong enough to have energy to spare — so I was on the menu.

I subsequently spoke with a Native American shaman who said this individual was one of the top dark shamans in the world. If such a shaman tries and fails to take the energy of another individual, under the shaman's code, that person becomes a candidate for apprenticeship, and the shaman teaches them all they know. The Native American shaman told me, "When he was trying to draw all the energy out of your heart, and suddenly the energy was released, it snapped back and caused tremendous pain in HIS heart." It was like he had a huge fish on his line, and the line snapped and hit him with a Divine force greater than his own will. He knew he was dealing with a force superior to his own.

Regardless of any shamanic explanation of how and why it happened, this much is clear. This experience changed my life forever in that I had direct experience of Source, beyond this world, beyond death, beyond time or space. Over the years, I came to understand that I co-created — with Source — this "initiation" so I could experience for myself life beyond the veil.

As a postscript to this story, I returned to Bali several years ago and found the shaman had died years before. The Temple of Death — that's what it was actually called — was closed to the public.

However, I had become friendly with the princess who controlled the land that had been the site of the temple. She and members of the family took me to that site, where we meditated and I did the Holoenergetic Forgiveness Process about the shamanic experience. The princess told me it was the most powerful meditation she had ever experienced. Although I had long since done the process for myself and released my own charge from the experience, this time there was a release of uncle into wholeness beyond time and space, from any judgments he had about himself.

So, why share this story?

To introduce you firsthand to the Game of Awakening.

We live in a civilization where the dominant paradigm is that only the material world is "real," and where everything we experience can be explained rationally. Because of this cultural conditioning, we become attached to the material conditions in our lives. We imagine our happiness and well-being comes from things and conditions outside us. Every time we hear a story or have an experience that cannot be explained by the laws of physical reality as we understand them, the grip of the ordinary world is weakened — and we potentially move closer to awakening to our essential nature and to who we really are.

As I said in the introduction, forgiveness is an important tool in the Game of Awakening because it frees us from the prison of the past.

There are many games we can play in life — the money game, the relationship game, the creativity game, the work game — and above and beyond all of these, the Game of Awakening is the Master Game. When we awaken to who we really are, all of the other games are put into perspective.

So … what is this Game of Awakening, and how do we play?

The Ocean of Awareness and the Game of Awakening

The Game of Awakening is about lifting the veils of the illusion of separation and recognizing wholeness as the inherent reality. There is only One. Not even the appearance of separation can be separate from the One. I could stop here because all else is just Oneness expressing as multiplicity.

One of the simplest yet most profound spiritual metaphors is that of the ocean and the waves as two ways of looking at the One.

As Thich Nhat Hanh said, "If a wave only sees its form, with its beginning and end, it will be afraid of birth and death. But if the wave sees that it is water, identifies itself with the water, then it will be emancipated from birth and death. Each wave is born and is going to die, but the water is free from birth and death."

We're all like waves in the Ocean of Awareness appearing to be separate.

First there was pure awareness, absolute Source. The wisdom traditions maintain that pure awareness interacted with itself creating a vibration called Consciousness — the first wave.

The First Wave — Consciousness
Awareness of Oneness

This first wave, pure awareness — aware of itself as consciousness — arises and is referred to as "I Am." The "I Am" is also known as "Being," as "I Exist," as "Radical Subject," as "That which looks" — the "I that looks with nothing to look at but itself." When "I Am" looked within, consciousness conscious of itself, it dissolved back into awareness as a wave dissolves in the ocean.

The Second Wave — Duality
The Appearance of Separation

When "I Am" looked out instead of within, and saw "I Am that I Am," this "I Am" consciousness interacted with itself creating the Second Wave, the Thinking Mind. The Thinking Mind divides the whole into self-other, observer-observed, subject-object duality, generating time/space and the multiplicity of forms.

The Third Wave — I/Me/Egoic Self
The Great Forgetting and the Cause of Suffering

To deepen the mystery, the Thinking Mind somehow folds upon itself and forgets completely that it is consciousness and then behaves as if it's independent from consciousness, forming the Third Wave — the "I/Me/Egoic Self." The Thinking Mind attaches its identity to this egoic self, which then compares and judges itself as "more than" or "less than" other selves, and projects the past into the future, bypassing the present.

The process of forgetting pure awareness is like the moon forgetting that it is reflecting the sun and seeing itself as the source of light.

This sense of separation from consciousness and the focus instead on the ever-changing forms that consciousness takes is at the core of all fear and suffering, including the fear of death. In my medical practice I observed that all suffering, distress, and many illnesses derive from this perceived sense of separation.

The Game of Awakening is the game of remembering the unity of pure awareness, from which everything comes and to which everything returns. Love is the reminder of that unity and the impulse to return to unity. In moving back from Third Wave to Second Wave to First Wave, we dissolve into ever-present Oneness. As we will see later, there are portals to Oneness that allow us to experience this Oneness while still in physical form.

Another way ever-present Oneness has been expressed in the Eastern traditions is that form is emptiness and emptiness appears as form, since both are composed of the same "substance" — consciousness itself. A classic analogy is that of the sand castle on the beach that is made of sand temporarily given form. Similarly, consciousness takes shape as form.

And even those forms that appear most unloving and fear based — war, rejection, resistance, violence, judgment, shame, anger, hatred — are really the one consciousness we call love disguised as separation. To paraphrase The Course in Miracles, all human behavior is either an expression of love or a call for love. While some would say these behaviors are an expression of our impulse to survive, ultimately none of us survives as a physical form — all the more reason to appreciate the formless, boundless context of loving consciousness. When we release our identification with fear-based separative forms and remember there is only one consciousness assuming many forms, we are home and we are free.

---

*Even those forms that appear most unloving and fear based
— war, rejection, resistance, violence, judgment, shame, anger,
hatred — are really the one consciousness we call love disguised as
separation.*

There is a natural relationship between Oneness and love because it is the nature of love to remember and seek unity. When love finds the unity it seeks, all further seeking stops. And when we awaken to the Oneness that is our inherent nature, we realize how much energy we have expended to maintain the illusion of separation. Whenever we feel tossed and thrown by the waves of circumstance and condition, it is helpful to remember the Ocean of Awareness, the ultimate reality.

And yet the illusion of separation is so much a part of our culture, our neurobiology, and such a big part of our self-identity that we find it hard to imagine who we would be or what we would do without these "precious" wounding stories.

As I have said, in my decades of practice I have found that all suffering, and most illness, can be traced back to this perceived sense of separation. There is a part of our self that we find too painful to hold in consciousness. So we separate from it. We disconnect from it, deny it, reject it, repress it, or project it onto others.

Early in our lives or perhaps in our mother's womb, something happened that caused us to feel we're not good enough or not loved, or that our existence is a mistake or a burden. In order to hold ourselves separate from this painful part, we simultaneously separate from others, from the world around us and most profoundly, from our spiritual essence — from Source.

Now, of course, distinctions are a necessary part of daily life. As we saw earlier in the Ocean of Awareness metaphor, in order for life to exist and reflect upon itself, awareness becomes aware of itself, creating consciousness, the first distinction. Then, consciousness divides itself into subject and object, creating duality, which is just the appearance of separation. Finally, consciousness forgets its Oneness, giving rise to the egoic experience of being a separate self — a stranger in a strange land.

In essence, the Game of Awakening is about forgetting and separating from Oneness and then remembering and returning to ever-present Oneness.

The diagram below shows Pure Awareness' cyclical journey from Oneness and back to Oneness, for the seeming purpose of experiencing duality and playing the Game of Awakening along the way. Through our soul, what we call the Aware Witness (covered in detail in chapter 6), we then dissolve back into the Ocean of Awareness. The Game of Awakening begins and ends with Awareness.

The Game of Awakening

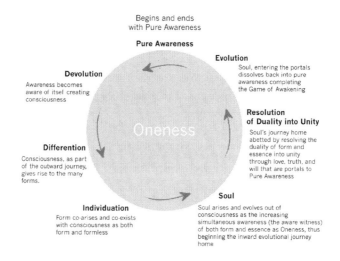

Begins and ends
with Pure Awareness

Pure Awareness

Evolution
Soul, entering the portals
dissolves back into pure
awareness completing
the Game of Awakening

Devolution
Awareness becomes
aware of itsef creating
consciousness

**Resolution
of Duality into Unity**
Soul's journey home
abetted by resolving the
duality of form and
essence into unity
through love, truth, and
will that are portals to
Pure Awareness

Differention
Consciousness, as part
of the outward journey,
gives rise to the many
forms.

Oneness

Soul
Soul arises and evolves out of
consciousness as the increasing
simultaneous awareness (the aware witness)
of both form and essence as Oneness, thus
beginning the inward evolutional journey
home

Individuation
Form co-arises and co-exists
with consciousness as both
form and formless

Prior to awakening, our tendency is to experience reality as the manifest forms, and not the unmanifest, formless consciousness that gives rise to the forms. In secular society, where only the material world is deemed "real," we are schooled in differentiation of one form from another. It's easy for most of us to recognize how we are different from other people and other creatures and mistake difference for separation. Remembering we are all sourced from the one consciousness appearing as different forms is the spiritual challenge of enlightenment. It is said that the forms are many, the essence is One.

Those initiatory drug experiences in the 1960s and 1970s temporarily liberated many individuals from the cultural filters that reinforced our separation from life. Perhaps that is something that indigenous people intrinsically knew and we have had to relearn. Experiencing the Holoenergetic Forgiveness Process can fully allow you to remember unity through unconditional love for yourself.

Remembering Unity serves to remind us of what we intrinsically know but have temporarily forgotten. It also allows us to reconnect and re-experience those "members" that have been dismembered (separated, cut off) by the limiting sense perceptions, beliefs and by the veils of our conditioned structures in consciousness.

We are inherently whole. Only the thinking mind dismembers us from our essence. The thinking mind divides observer and observed creating subject/object and time/space duality. It is the "function" of love to make us aware of wholeness. It does not bring us into wholeness because we are already always whole. Through love we can awaken to Oneness.

We are inherently whole. Only the thinking mind dismembers us from our essence.

Love Is the Impulse Toward Unity

Love is one of the most commonly used yet one of the least clearly defined words in our language, perhaps because love can mean or refer to so many different things:

I love pizza.

I love my country.

I love my brothers and sisters.

I love my lover.

I love God.

In Sanskrit, there are ninety-six terms for love. Each representation of love reflects a deep appreciation for and connection with someone or something — with an individual or individuals, with Spirit, with beloved objects, ideas, and places.

Let's consider that commonly uttered phrase, "I love you." When we tell our loved ones, "I love you," what are we really saying?

Look at these three words: "I love you:" subject (I) verb (love) object (you). What if the distinction or separation between subject/object were just a perceptual illusion created by the thinking mind and its extension, the senses? What if subject/object, I/you, observer and observed were not ever really separate, but only appeared to be?

What would be left of "I love you" if, at a deeper level, there was no separate "I" or "you"? What would be left is love — the thoughts, feelings and a felt sense of connectedness or oneness called love.

Having worked with and experienced the healing power of love — as described in greater depth in my book Healing with Love — I utilized an operational definition that includes the many "flavors" of love.

Love is the urge to merge with the object of that love, evoking a felt sense of unity.

Love is the awareness of connectedness and the impulse toward unity.

Love is being aware of One as many, and the many as One.

This "unconditional" love is more than the sentimental love of romantic movies and far transcends the word we use so casually. Whether we love sunsets, or Paris in the springtime, it's still a pale reflection of that larger impulse toward unity. You CAN feel connection with some food you're eating, with a special person or persons, with a cherished activity, with Source. When we feel these connections in varying degrees, we are experiencing, in that moment, a sense of unconditional love — a love that resolves duality into Unity.

Remember those bacteria from the introduction? In order to unconditionally accept those bacteria enough for them to respond to my intention that they slow their growth, I had to "merge" with them at the level of consciousness, theirs and mine. So when we focus on the object of our love we want to merge with it — be it a food we love, a dear friend, or a lover. To the extent that we love, we come into resonant harmony with the object of our love.

Whatever we feel love for, we want to merge with and become resonantly one with. And ultimately, we want to become one with the Divine, which I call "the vertical aspect" of love. In the realm of duality and form, this desire for oneness is expressed as a feeling of relatedness, of connectedness, which I call "the horizontal aspect" of love.

Love and Resonance

Love expresses and experiences itself as both passion and peace, cyclically and simultaneously unfolding in the totality of being. The "medium" for our passionate and peaceful intentions is "resonance," which is one of the keys to healing. The classic example of resonance involves two tuning forks, each having the same natural frequency, in tune with one another. If you strike one tuning fork tuned to A and put it next to another A tuning fork, it will induce a vibration in the other. If you put that same vibrating tuning fork next to a B or C tuning fork, it will not vibrate. There is no resonance. Only similars vibrate.

We can't equate love with resonance per se because, for example, if you have unresolved anger and you walk into a room where there are angry people, you might get angry at them or with them. That anger is activated through resonance with the anger within you. So resonance by itself is not an example of love. However, when you are loving, resonance is always present. In other words, resonance is necessary but not sufficient for healing with love.

Love doesn't "create" unity because Oneness already IS. The function of love is to remember Oneness. That is what the Game of Awakening is all about. We live in a world of apparent separation, and love reminds us that there is only One appearing as many. It reconnects us with our missing "members" — whether those members be fragmented parts of ourselves, others we feel alienated from, or our own connection with Source. Love "awakens" us to the unity that is ever present, and brings back the members that appeared separate but never were.

Love doesn't "create" unity because Oneness already IS. Love "awakens" us to the unity that is ever present.

The cycle of peace and passion is another rhythm of life — like night and day, action and non-action, rest and activity — duality in the greater context of unity. Simultaneously and cyclically, our soul seeks peace and passion. Passion moves us while peace stills us. Without passion, there would be no action and no movement. We are both the passion and peace of love, love's form and formlessness, the delicious drop of love that dissolves into the unknowable, unspeakable One, only to reappear as the love dance of Unity.

Ultimately, love seeks unity. When love becomes the unity it seeks, all desire, searching, seeking, passion and movement ceases. What remains is aware stillness; only stillness abides.

We have all experienced timeless moments when all movement stops. Can you recall a situation when time stopped for you, no past, no future — only the eternal present? Was it looking into the eyes of a child or a lover? Was it being in nature? A sunset? A full moon? These moments of stillness are portals to the eternal. When time stands still, we experience freedom in its truest sense as pure awareness.

Forgiving Dissolves the Veils of Separation

As mentioned, when I started exploring healing and forgiveness in my practice selectively with patients, I noticed that almost all the suffering, distress, and many illnesses were associated with a perceived sense of separation — from others, from our environment, or most importantly, from our spiritual nature. Specifically, I noticed a tendency to "dissociate" or deny a part of oneself from an experience or wound too painful to hold in consciousness. Often this wounding came in early childhood, and sometimes it even went back to being in the womb. It's not uncommon for people to pick up feelings from their mother or father or the collective consciousness while in this precognitive state and then attribute these to themselves. For example, "I'm not good enough," "I'm a mistake," "My father wanted a boy, and I'm a girl."

Sometimes they sense the fear the mother has about her own capability to care for her infant, particularly if they are the firstborn. Again, because they are precognitive, these are feelings without language. If they did have words, the words might say, "How am I going to survive if she feels that way?" or "There must be something wrong with ME."

We are, of course, rarely conscious of holding these early beliefs and decisions about how the world is and how things are. And yet, they are so often at the root of our problems, our suffering, and most of our illnesses. These emotional wounds initiate our sense of separation from others, from our environment, and ultimately, from our essential nature.

Forgiving yourself dissolves the veils that obscure your inner light — your loving presence. What are these veils of separation? What are these structures in consciousness called the conditioned mind? Unconscious identification with your mind-made self veils you from your loving presence as: thoughts, feelings, sense perceptions, as your story, illness, pain, suffering and loss, your attachments and aversions, your judgments of others and especially of yourself. So forgiveness is about letting go, about releasing, about dissolving these veils of the conditioned mind.

To forgive is to heal the separation from your inner light — your loving presence — by dissolving the veils of separation.

Forgiving yourself is one of the most powerful ways to unveil your essential nature to let your inner light shine. And through for-

giveness, we experience freedom, truth, love and peace. You may ask
yourself where is this freedom, truth, love and peace? It is within.
It's about what is happening inside of you, the forgiver. So forgiveness is not about another, although that is the common misperception. Perpetrators need to forgive themselves. However, everything
is non-locally connected, so when you release them through forgiveness, they frequently feel it. Another way to say this is that, since we
are all interrelated, actually entangled at the level of consciousness,
when you change, the relationship changes.

Forgiveness is about letting go. Letting go of what? It is about
releasing attachment to the past, and attachment to resentments,
grudges and anger. It's letting go of attachment to judgment, blame,
shame, guilt, suffering and loss, victim-victimizer perspective, and
especially identifying with the story. It's letting go of the story of
abandonment, betrayal, loss, and the need to control through continued judgment and anger.

Fundamentally, forgiveness is letting go of the charge around
the memory so that upon recalling what happened in the past, there
is no longer an emotional reaction, just the memory. Now you are
free — free to love and free to be.

Forgiving heals the separation from your inner light — your loving presence — by dissolving the veils of conditioned perception
and belief. When you release the identification with the story, when
you release the illusion that who you are is the story with its experiences and memories, when you really release the illusion, what
remains is love.

Although we commonly think about forgiveness with regard to
other people, it requires no one but yourself. When Pope John Paul II
publicly forgave Mehmet Ali Agca, the man who tried to assassinate
him, the Pope freed himself. Forgiving is not the same as forgetting.
It is doubtful the Pope "forgot" that this man had tried to kill him.
However, in forgiving the man he released any emotional charge he
may have had around the memory. As we will see when we discuss
the biology of forgiveness, when we release the charge around painful memories, our body chemistry and physiology actually change.

The act of genuine forgiveness frees us from bondage — from resentment, judgment, blame, or wanting — to see that person pay a price, to be held accountable. Accountability is the domain of criminal law, civil law, and Divine Law. Your choice is to free yourself by letting all of that go. Let go of the need to control through holding on to your story about the situation, let go of your attachment to the story, let go of using it as an excuse to avoid growing. By forgiving, you allow yourself to evolve into the fullness of who you really are.

Giving Ourselves Freedom

It takes energy to hold on — to a grievance, a story, anything that happened. When genuine forgiveness finally occurs, there is a huge sigh of relief, and what you have is freedom. You have freed your past and your future into the present.

And you have freed happiness from being attached to any condition. Pleasure and pain are part of life, generally as signals to "stop" or "go." They ebb and flow, come and go, and when we allow them to move in that way, we are in the flow of life. When we hold on to pleasure — or seek to hold off pain — when we are attached to things being a certain way, our happiness becomes conditional. That's when "problems" appear as something we have that we don't want, or something we don't have that we do want.

Forgiveness detaches us from our attachments and gives us the freedom to BE with life, moment to moment. Please note the distinction between connection and attachment. We can be connected to an individual, a place, an idea, and anything we resonate with. Connection becomes attachment when that relationship becomes conditional — I cannot live without that person, I MUST have that house, things have to be A CERTAIN WAY for me to be happy. When we identify with thoughts, feelings, beliefs, objects, individuals, we forget the unconditioned nature of life. We release attachment by remembering and identifying with Source, with stillness. Source is everywhere yet is no thing. You cannot attach yourself to it because there is nothing to attach to. Remembering this can spontaneously dissolve attachment into Oneness / stillness / Source.

Forgiveness detaches us from our attachments and gives us the freedom to BE with life, moment to moment.

The revered sage from India, Nisargadatta said, "When I recognize that I am nothing, that is WISDOM. When I recognize that I am everything, that is LOVE. My life flows between the two."

He could have added: when I recognize that I am nothing, that is PEACE. The Everything is fullness, vibrancy, radiance, energy, passion. And the Nothing is emptiness, stillness, peace.

Forgiveness frees us from the prison of conditioned reactivity to experience both aliveness and peace. Freedom implies the ability to choose, and paradoxically choosing WHAT IS in this moment is a direct path to freedom. The first liberating choice is to accept what is as being so. As the song goes, freedom's just another word for nothing left to lose. When you need nothing, you have nothing to lose and nothing to gain. You "die before dying," meaning that you are complete with life exactly as it is this moment. You are free to experience this moment without future expectation or attachment to the past. The "I" and "me" disappear — no subject, no object — and all that remains is love. Like the Buddha, you are "awake."

Acceptance Liberates Us

Acceptance is an important first step in forgiving. When we accept a condition, we liberate the energy we had used to deny, repress or project. Acceptance of the truth allows the painful feelings to come up for healing and release. Finally, when we unconditionally love and accept ourselves as we are, we are free to simply Be. So it isn't mere acceptance that brings freedom; it's acceptance of the truth of what is and the truth of what we are feeling. Love is the unconditional acceptance of what is.

For forgiveness to be complete, and for the conditioning to be released, there are three steps:

1. Accept the truth of what is or what appears to be, and in particular accept the emotional content of what is or what is perceived to be.

2. Free yourself from the emotional charge of the past.

3. Unconditionally love and accept yourself as you are.

Step one allows you to be present with what is.

Step two frees you from the past.

Step three opens to loving yourself as you are.

You are now free to Be who you truly are. So, forgiving is for giving yourself love and freedom.

As life unfolds in complexity, it is also true that all roads lead home, back to the One. A direct way "home" is through the portal of forgiveness. When you've learned this process of shifting from contraction to expansion to transcendence, your life will never be the same.

Given the extraordinary benefits of forgiveness, why don't we forgive? In the next chapter, we will learn how to cultivate our willingness to forgive and allow our inner light and loving awareness to shine forth. Then we step off the game board of the Game of Awakening — at one with Source.

As the great sage Ramana Maharshi said as he was dying and his disciples were lamenting his death, "Where can I go?"

LOVE, TRUTH, AND WILL

Love seeks unity as knowing seeks truth. When love becomes the unity it seeks, all desire, searching, seeking, and movement cease. Desire always implies movement, either toward an object of desire or, if an aversion, a movement away from it. So, when love finally becomes the unity it seeks, all movement, all seeking stops. Love becomes stillness.

Similarly, once knowing merges with truth, seeking and desiring to know ceases. In that timeless moment, only aware stillness abides. Truth becomes stillness, the same stillness that love brings. So ultimately, love and truth are one and the same — two portals leading to the One.

The search for truth is searching for love because the ultimate truth is the Unity of everything and nothing.

The truth shall set you free ... be still and be God.

Ultimately will seeks Oneness with Divine Will. Initially, personal will seeks unity with the intended outcome. When the outcome that it seeks is realized, all seeking, all movement temporarily ends. Out of this stillness, a sense of short-lived peace or joy arises.

When personal will is surrendered to Divine Will, all seeking stops. What remains is stillness. Not my will, but Thy Will be done.

This boundless, indescribable stillness, when expressed in language as experience, has many labels:

Love

Peace

Freedom

Joy

Oneness

Unity

Wholeness

God

Source

Pure awareness

Grace

Love, truth, and will are expressions of Source flowing through human existence.

It's like the one light refracted into love, truth, and will so that Source can express and experience itself.

CHAPTER 2

FORGIVENESS — WHAT IT IS AND WHAT IT IS NOT

You need to not aspire for or get any new state. Get rid of your present thoughts, that is all.
— *Ramana Maharshi*

It's not what happens that creates our experience of the event, it's our perception and interpretation of it.
— *Leonard Laskow*

Forgiveness may be the most powerful tool in the toolkit for those of us willing to play the Game of Awakening. And yet, for many it is the most difficult thing to do. Why is that?

For some, it means looking at something deemed "unlovable." Many of us — regardless of how difficult or easy our lives have been — have had some experience, some condition, or some situation that we've thought of as "unforgivable."

Throughout history, humans have done horrific things to other humans, and these perpetrations tend to harden into "stories" that each generation seems to build one more "story" high. The greater the perpetration, the more righteously people hold on to being wronged. As a child and teenager growing up in the wake of the Holocaust, I still remember the slogan that most Jewish people accepted without questioning: We will never forgive, we will never forget.

Here we are years later with the conflict transferred to the Middle East, and the "promised land" now under siege as well. A Holy War in the Holy Land ...

Most people miss the sad irony in this oxymoron. It might just be the power of forgiveness that holds the key to unlock us from the prison of the past. And it's the misperceptions about the nature of forgiveness — which we will address shortly — that keep people on the battlefield of perpetration and retaliation.

So, what is forgiveness ... and what is it not?

The purpose of forgiveness is to release attachment to the past so that we are free to live and love in the present. We practice forgiveness through the truthful acceptance of what has been and what we felt, in the field of unconditioned love. When we release attachment to the past and the emotional charge associated with it, we have the freedom to love ourselves fully and completely, without condition.

The purpose of forgiveness is to release attachment to the past so that we are free to live and love in the present.

Notice we use the term, "unconditioned" rather than the more common "unconditional." There are two reasons. First, the phrase "unconditional love" has been used so commonly and freely that it has become almost a cliché, meaning that it's a catch phrase that has little transformational impact. I prefer "unconditioned" because as a practicing physician, I've come to recognize how many of our physical conditions are due to our emotional and mental conditioning.

To me, the term "unconditioned" transcends the conditioned structures or veils in consciousness that filter our perceptions of reality. It represents a state of awakened awareness, the quiet voice that says, "I am more than my body, my mind, and the conditions in my life." Unconditioned love is a love with no judgments, no attachment to outcome, a love without condition, reason, or cause, beyond time and space, even beyond understanding.

As a brief yet important aside here, I sometimes make a further distinction between "unconditioned" and "non-conditioned" love. Unconditioned love has a focus, a vector, and an object; it can be directed toward someone or something. When not directed or focused, I call the same love non-conditioned love. Non-conditioned love is radiant like the sun and has no focus; it shines on all alike. You can have both unconditioned and non-conditioned love simultaneously. You can also have one or the other. Both unconditioned and non-conditioned love are reflections and fractals of Source.

When I refer to fractals, I am talking about the geometric patterns that repeat themselves in nature at increasing levels of complexity. There seems to be growth when there is a fractal … the veiny patterns in leaves are repeated in the branches of trees, so that the entire forest is a fractal of one leaf. And yet, although the form may increase in complexity, it is still born of the same Oneness. Leaf or forest, molehill or mountain, all come from the same Source. It's almost as if each relationship contributes to the new form. When we become aware of a relationship through unconditioned love, we become aware of the seeming other as an expression of the One, in a new form or variety. That is why I call love the Divine fractal. Through love's expression, beyond the comprehension of the thinking mind, the Divine continues to creatively express its oneness.

Before we scale the transcendent heights of love without condition, let's explore the benefits of forgiving and the often misunderstood idea of "forgiveness."

Benefits of Forgiving

Feeling loved and loving
Feeling good enough
Feeling and being connected and aligned with Source
Feeling and being more related to the world and other people
Physical, emotional, and spiritual healing
Feeling and being energized, vital, alive
Fulfilling and joyful relationships
Clarity about life and life purpose
Joy and lasting happiness

3 Misconceptions about Forgiveness

If forgiveness has so many irresistible benefits, why do we so often resist it?

There are many reasons, but the most obvious ones have to do with three common misconceptions about forgiveness:

    1. Forgiving means condoning the harm others have done.

    2. To forgive means to forget.

    3. Forgiveness is about another or others.

So … if those beliefs aren't true, then what is true?

To Forgive Is NOT to Condone

The most common reason given for not forgiving is: If I forgive _____ for doing _____ that would mean I am condoning that behavior.

Merriam-Webster dictionary defines condone as "to forgive or approve (something that is considered wrong); to allow (something that is considered wrong) to continue."

Here is where the dictionary misses the mark when it equates "forgiving" with "approving." Consider that when Jesus said, "Forgive them Father because they know not what they do," he wasn't saying, "And I APPROVE of what they did."

Forgiveness is entirely different from approval. Also, forgiveness has nothing to do with allowing the offensive behavior to continue.

True forgiveness offers a subtle yet key distinction between accepting that something happened ... and accepting that something should have happened. It happened, and there is no way to make it "un-happen." The ultimate focus of forgiveness extends beyond accepting what happened to releasing identification with the past. Through the release of emotional past attachment, we release ourselves from the pain in the past and free ourselves to experience the present and future anew. That's why I say forgiving is "for giving love, and for giving freedom."

With the bacteria in the laboratory, I unconditionally accepted their existence yet sought to change their behavior (i.e., growth rate). When we forgive an individual, we allow their right to "be"; we don't condone their right to "do" what we have deemed wrongful and hurtful.

Forgiveness in this regard frees both the "victim" and the perpetrator. The perpetrator is freed from the expectation that they will do the same thing in the future. The victim is freed from the prison of conditioned reactivity — meaning, they are no longer "locked in" to their pain around the incident. They are free, free to choose something other than blame and anger with its concomitant emotional charge.

Most importantly, forgiveness is for freeing ourselves. In doing so, we create space for a new relationship with the forgiven party to emerge — or not. Quite often, the forgiven individual DOES show up differently, as we will discover later. This can be considered a "collateral benefit" of forgiveness.

Again — and this is important enough to reiterate — forgiving is not condoning what has happened. It simply releases us from the prison of conditioned reactivity.

Forgiving is not condoning what has happened. It simply releases
us from the prison of conditioned reactivity.

The Biology of Forgiveness

That common phrase, "forgive and forget" does us a disservice by linking the two. The latest discoveries in epigenetic biology offer us a more accurate and helpful understanding: "Forgive and remember differently."

In working with clients using the Holoenergetic Forgiveness Process, I've found that the emotional charge associated with painful or stressful events can be altered or even released completely. Transmuting the pain has nothing whatsoever to do with forgetting, just with how and where these memories are held.

Recent neurologic research suggests that short-term memory goes through a molecular process called "consolidation" during which it is converted, under certain circumstances, into long-term memories. The process of converting short-term memories to long-term ones is enhanced by stress hormones, which alert a part of the midbrain called the amygdala, the brain's emotional control center. The amygdala is activated either by stress hormones or those associated with love and caring. You probably can't even imagine how many events in your life you have forgotten. Notice however, how many of the events you do recall are associated with either contractive or expansive emotions. That's because recall is tethered to emotions.

Exciting new research suggests that original memories can be changed or reconsolidated. For example, when rats were given an electric shock at the exact moment a sound was played, the rats formed a memory that linked the sound to fear. For a memory to be consolidated from short term to long term — from unstable to stable — it undergoes a process called protein synthesis. The researchers theorized that during this unstable memorizing period, the memories could be reconsolidated. They injected a drug that stopped the protein synthesis in the amygdala of the rat. When the sound was played after that, the rats no longer reacted with fear to hearing the sound alone.

The implications are this: Reactivating a memory temporarily returns it to an unstable state, providing an opportunity to reconsolidate the memory. If the reactivation occurs in a loving field, the memory can be favorably reconsolidated. That's why the Holoenergetic Forgiveness Process works so well. It allows us to remember the experience without the painful emotional charge.

Other researchers working with people who experienced a traumatic event injected propranolol, a drug that reduces anxiety, to see if it could stop long-term traumatic memories. Propranolol blocks the action of adrenaline, a stress hormone known to strengthen emotionally significant memories. Using this approach, researchers were able to reduce symptoms by fifty percent. The scientists tentatively concluded that long-term memory appears to reside in a part of the midbrain called the hippocampus. However, the emotional trauma of that memory seems to be located in the amygdala. Current research is focused on being able to target and reconsolidate just the fear part of the memory located in the amygdala, which leaves the details of the memory intact. In other words, there is less charge associated with the memory, less physiologic response to the memory.

As an obstetrician, I've noticed that even though childbirth is generally associated with pain, most mothers recalling the experience don't have a contractive emotional charge. My sense is that this may be due to the hormones and neuropeptides present at birth — oxytocin, prolactin, dopamine, atrial natriuretic peptide plus endorphins — which neutralize the adrenaline's impact on the amygdala. These hormones of birth are also the hormones produced by love. In fact, the heart is a major producer of oxytocin and atrial natriuretic peptide. Perhaps this is nature's way of physiologically assuring the presence of a loving, nurturing mother to receive her baby.

What I've noticed clinically is that by activating the memory of a stressful event in the presence of or immediately followed by feelings that evoke love, the stressful emotional charge is neutralized even though the memory remains. This is what the Holoenergetic Forgiveness Process does so effectively. It allows us to "keep" the experience as something we can learn from, yet frees us from the physiologic and psychological burdens of carrying the emotional charge. The quality of our lives depends on the amount of charge we carry. To live freely, we need to be free of reactive conditioning expressed as emotional charge.

When you forgive fully, you open a portal to ever-present Oneness. Once charge is released, you are free to experience "what is" directly instead of through the filter of past conditioning. Your quality of life dramatically improves and you are free to be who you truly are.

Often when people are initially exposed to the idea of Oneness, they make that unity their pursuit. Therein lies an irony. There is no need to pursue "oneness." Oneness is already ever present, so it isn't a place to "get to." The very pursuit of Oneness keeps us separate, temporarily disconnecting us from the Oneness that is always present.

So, forgiveness is a major portal to unconditioned self-acceptance and love for yourself, allowing you freedom to be who you really are. Now is the time for giving yourself love, freedom, and peace. Choose now to release attachment to story, anger, shame, blame, guilt, judgment, and control that separate you from your essential nature.

And if you choose not to forgive?

Some of the consequences that I've seen in people who are unwilling or unable to forgive include:

Stress, nightmares, and sleeplessness

A diminished sense of self-worth, lack of self-esteem

Strong feelings of guilt or shame

Difficulty controlling anger

Compromised immune system, diminished endocrine function, which predisposes one to chronic illnesses, such as: rheumatoid arthritis, fibromyalgia, diabetes, cancer, and heart disease along with skin disorders, chronic fatigue, asthma, a variety of headaches, neck and back pain, and difficulty in maintaining intimate relationships.

So, forgiveness means accepting what happened without condoning it and, through the Holoenergetic Forgiveness Process, remembering the incident in such a way that releases emotional charge and attachment to the past — consequently freeing us to be healthier and more loving.

And that brings us to the third misconception about forgiveness — that it somehow requires another person be involved.

Forgiveness Is in the "I" of the Beholder

The third misconception about forgiveness is that there has to be some other person in the picture who is there to either ask for forgiveness or accept your forgiveness. As we have suggested earlier, the act of forgiveness is to free oneself from the prison of reactivity. No one else need be involved.

Are you waiting for someone else to forgive you for some real or perceived transgression? You may have a long wait, particularly if the other party is no longer alive. The important thing to remember is the attachment to this past situation is inside you and located in structures in consciousness you hold in place. You and only you can release them, and now is the time.

The attachment to the past situation is inside you, and only you can release it.

Forgiveness is not contingent upon what another person does or does not do. We hold the key to our own freedom. No one else need be involved. Forgiving isn't condoning, and it isn't forgetting. And yet ... still there may be resistance.

Why is that?

It is our attachment to separation.

Let's just say we are of two minds — the small, local, ego mind and the Aware Witness, which resonates with our uniqueness and unity simultaneously, also known as our soul.

The Aware Witness and the Little Me

If you've ever said that you're "of two minds" about something, you're probably right. As human beings, we express both the more human "doing" part of us (the smaller ego-based "me"), and the being part of us (the larger part that is fully aligned with Source). Neither of these is to be judged "right" or "wrong"; they are both aspects through which the Aware Witness is attempting to find balance between doing and being. When we are operating from the Aware Witness, we are better able to navigate lovingly through life.

What we call the "ego" is a set of conditioned structures in consciousness that affect our thoughts, our feelings, and our sense perceptions. Our conscious mind then identifies with these structures in consciousness, thereby creating a false sense of self, called "I" / "me," which then divides the world into "me/mine" and other or "not me/not mine." This false sense of self then struggles to maintain this illusion of separation, as it seeks to control "what's mine" and reject, resist, deny, or control what's "not mine."

This persistent process of grasping and resisting is what many humans would call "life" — and yet, these limited responses are merely the shadow of who we really are and can be. It is a projection of fear, a primal force that is activated when we feel our survival is threatened — even when it isn't. All of that energy is expended, just to protect and preserve an illusion.

The ego — the agent of form-based consciousness — sees itself as only this physical form and personality. By adding more things — and then defending or protecting these structures — the ego, or little "me," imagines it is enhancing its survival and achieving happiness. However, as many wise teachers have said, "Nothing will make you happy." What they mean is "no thing will make you happy."

Happiness is not of the world of things.

Until we realize that all forms are derivative of consciousness, the ego will dominate and use all the familiar mechanisms to maintain this false sense of self: denial, suppression, repression, projection, withdrawal, blame, guilt, shame, punishment, judgment, and misperception. By totally identifying with thoughts, beliefs and concepts, with feelings and sense perceptions, and with the past, the egoic or psychological self creates the structures in consciousness that veil our inner light and separate us from our essential nature.

Forgiveness is a way to release the illusion of separation and experience our essential nature once again. And that, paradoxically, is another source of resistance to forgiving. If we forgave, the ego would have one less story to protect, one less illusion to live by. In releasing these stories and attachments, these long-held interpretations of reality, the ego self feels its very existence threatened — hence the resistance.

Forgiveness is a way to release the illusion of separation and experience our essential nature once again.

Sometimes in the wake of forgiveness, there is a greater awakening in the form of transcendent awareness of who we are beyond form and ego. While this doesn't happen all the time, transcendence can be the collateral benefit of the Holoenergetic Forgiveness Process.

Awareness and Differentiation

A key to understanding how and why forgiveness works is this. At the root of everything, there is pure Awareness, and all else de-

rives from awareness being aware of itself. It may not be a coinci-
dence that the first game babies love to play is peekaboo — now you
see it, now you don't. In order for awareness to be aware of itself, it
separates into observer and observed, creating duality and the world
of form.

Without "differentiation" and duality, there would be no movement, no contrast — no game, and no world. So now think of your
favorite sports team and your favorite players. In order to have a
game worth watching, there has to be an opposing team — something to push up against and overcome. You have only to look at the
faces of competitive athletes in action to see that they are intently
focused on their game. On the field of play, it's the ONLY thing
happening.

But when the game is over, what happens then?

The athletes take off their uniforms, they shower, and they go
home to their "other" lives. The most successful among them are the
ones who are able to play all out, and then "leave the game on the
field." They may even go out for a beer with opposing players.

So what's the point?

The point is, our ego is the "player" we put on the playing field
to play this game of apparent separation so that awareness can have
the full experience of being aware. When we allow ourselves to experience the release of forgiveness, we liberate a huge amount of
pent-up energy. We leave the game on the field and experience a moment or even an extended period of time, beyond time, where pure
awareness shines through. Then once again, we "suit up" for the
game revitalized and refreshed. Or, finally, we see the game for what
it is and step off the game board entirely — at peace — utterly free.

Pure awareness is the same in all of us. It is the mind-made
structures in consciousness that act like a prism refracting the pure
light of awareness into multiple frequencies of color. When awareness is aware of itself and turns outward, it creates the world of
relativity, multiplicity, and duality — the world of differentiation.
When awareness identifies with its content or form, that is called
ego. When it transcends the identification with the ego, it realizes

its essential nature, yet again.

What differentiates the master teachers from the aspirants is their ability to transcend the little-me mind. The masters simultaneously shift into and abide as Unity Consciousness. As we mentioned earlier, unconditioned love is the universal harmonic. Its "tone" resonantly returns us to Source. As the absolute becomes relative through the mind, so love in the heart facilitates the shift into unity. Forgiving is one profound way to predispose the shift.

When forgiveness is unconditioned and entered into fully, it transcends all conditions. When we have exhausted all "rational" reasons for not forgiving, we are left with a choice. Which self — the little me, or the Aware Witness— will prevail?

We'd all love to say, "Why the Aware Witness, of course!"

Except that, when we are faced with circumstances where everything tells us we've been "wronged," our egoic selves desperately want to be right about being wronged! How do we know we've been wronged? Our perceptions tell us so. And ... as we will learn in the next chapter, our perceptions and actual reality might be two different things. This is not to say that the hurtful and damaging things we've experienced are merely the creation of the egoic self. They really happened. Forgiveness is the way to neutralize the emotional charge and give us access to our Aware Witness.

Judgment, Discernment, and Treasured Wounds

Whenever judgment arises, resistance to forgiving comes with it. That's why it might seem that forgiveness is the ultimate test of the power of love. What we judge most harshly, we deem unworthy of love. Of course, there is a functional aspect of judgment that we call "discernment." If our ancestors hadn't learned to discern nutritious from poisonous plants, we wouldn't be here now. Our ability to navigate life successfully depends on our ability to distinguish what is healthy for us and what isn't.

Judgment has a lot to do with those two highly charged words, "good" and "bad." There is finality to a judgment, as we put someone or something into a box — or a prison cell. Judgment says something is intrinsically good or bad at the level of being. Had I been judgmental about the cancer cells in the laboratory, I would have charged them as guilty. I never would have had the experience of accepting them as they are, blending with them, and guiding them to return to the natural order and harmony of their pre-hyperactive state.

Judgment often has an emotional charge around it that creates separation from something or someone forever, for all time. Discernment is situational and involves a certain neutrality, a lack of attachment. As author Ken Keyes suggested, we can choose to evolve our addictions into preferences. We may, for example, prefer a high-calorie dessert in some situations and not others. Rather than judge these desserts as "bad," we suspend judgment and discern when having the dessert is appropriate, and when it is not.

So next time we are making a "judgment call," notice if it is a categorical condemnation or really a "discernment call" in service to our well-being, here and now.

In the early 1940s, the theologian Reinhold Niebuhr popularized the Serenity Prayer: "God grant me the serenity to accept the things I cannot change; courage to change the things I can; and wisdom to know the difference."

And yet, how often do we mentally obsess over what cannot be changed, expending valuable energy that could be used to change what we CAN change?

What keeps us on this field of misspent energy — not to mention frustration, grief, and suffering — is our ego's addiction to our story, particularly stories that involve a "treasured wound." As suggested earlier, many people have justified their own perpetrations by pointing to what has been done to them. Others have justified what they HAVEN'T accomplished in their life by pointing to some early wounding incident.

Consider the paradox in the phrase, "treasured wound." Why

would a wound be treasured? What could be valuable about it? Besides being the perfect excuse to justify present shortcomings, it is the IDENTIFICATION with the story that blurs the distinction between the Aware Witness we really are, and the "little me" personality we imagine ourselves to be. Who would I be without my story? What meaning would my life have without this treasured wound?

This is no idle question. In preparing for the freedom that forgiveness promises, are you ready for that freedom? Are you ready and willing to be someone and something other than that limiting story?

On a more subtle level, think about the "juice" we get from negativity — from gossip, from commiserating friends, from secret fantasies of revenge or retribution. Why do people watch reality TV shows about dysfunctional people? Why do they listen to opposing political commentators that make them furious? Why do some of us "love to hate"?

Are we willing to release these habitual perception and energy patterns? Are we ready to have well-being and peace of mind?

Treasured wounds can take other forms as well, such as attachment to long-departed loved ones — or wrongs done generations ago. We may still be carrying that banner for "our people" — whoever those people might be.

There is no judgment about any of these attachments. As part of the human condition (i.e., human conditioning), we learn as children when we hurt ourselves and start crying that we can get attention from those big, powerful folks — and maybe even use that wound to get what we want. However, as part of human evolution — individual and collective — we eventually learn that staying weak and helpless ultimately has no enduring benefit.

Also, there are those who learn that their illness or physical disability will get them special attention. So they habitually manifest illness (or hypochondria) in later life.

Before we move on to even more subtle blockages to forgiveness and awakening — like mistaking perceptions for reality — let's consider a few more habits, qualities, traits, and ways of being that keep us in the illusion of separation.

Guilt. Guilt might originate with something harmful you've done, but it can readily rigidify into anger turned inward. It may seem odd to associate guilt with anger, but consider that when one is caught, there is anger at being caught. Since there was likely a perpetration, you don't feel right having this anger, so it gets turned inward.

Shame. Shame goes even deeper than guilt because rather than it being about something you did, shame is about who you are. Guilt might say, "I did something bad." Shame says, "I'm a bad person." All the more reason to shift to the Game of Awakening so that we recognize the being we truly are.

Self-Pity. This desire to bewail one's own condition thinly disguises a desire to punish oneself — which is often really a desire to hurt or punish someone else by punishing oneself. This is closely related to the martyr who suffers to obtain sympathy.

Fear. When we fear for our own safety or well-being, we go into protection mode. We are reluctant to confront anything — a situation we feel has hurt us or the potential hurt of uncovering a perpetration. Fear is accompanied by the experience of contraction and separation. While the flash of fear that warns us of an immediate danger is biologically necessary for survival, if we habitually experience chronic fear and anxiety, we project conditions and situations from the past onto the future.

Doubt. Shakespeare called doubt the greatest traitor of them all. Doubt shakes our self-confidence and our faith in the unseen, which is, as we are learning, where our essential nature resides.

Do you notice something that all of these limiting ways of behaving have in common? They are all about the past. Eckhart Tolle says, in the present there are no problems, just what is. Freedom is about being in the present. When we free ourselves from the past through forgiveness, we are present as presence. Life is new to us, moment by moment.

When we free ourselves from the past through forgiveness, we are
present as presence. Life is new to us, moment by moment.

Alignment with your soul and essential nature allows you to release your attachment and identifications with treasured tragedies
and stories. When you establish your connection to what you really are, these lesser roles and stories fall into proper perspective.
Yes, you will still be someone's child and possibly someone's spouse
or parent. Yes, you will still remember your experiences. You will
still have a history and memories, both pleasant and unpleasant.
You might still identify with your profession or passion, or wear a
T-shirt or button proclaiming a political position. The difference is,
you won't BE any of those things. You are the Aware Witness and
not subject to the objects in your life.

EXPERIENCING LOVING PRESENCE — THE CON-
SCIOUS HEART FOCUS

The purpose of the Conscious Heart Focus is:

- To evoke inner peace, centeredness, and expanded awareness
- To generate harmonious and coherent heart energies
- To invoke and evoke loving, healing presence

To begin the process, make yourself comfortable. Gently close
your eyes and allow yourself to begin to relax.

One of the best ways to relax is to become aware of your breathing, so allow yourself now to notice your breathing.

- Become aware that when you are breathing in, you are breathing in and when you are breathing out, you are breathing out.
- If other thoughts, feelings, or sensations come to mind, gently but firmly bring your awareness back to your breath ...
- Now shift your attention to the center of your chest, your
  heart center. Slowly breathe in and out, as if through the
  center of your chest, for at least three breaths.
- In this peaceful and relaxed heart space, recall a wonder-

ful heart-opening experience. Allow yourself to feel these heart-full feelings now — perhaps feelings of love, caring, gratitude, aliveness, joy, deep inner peace, or flowing in the moment.

- Your experience may be in nature, in solitude, with another, or others.
- Allow yourself to really feel these feelings while continuing to breathe in and out through the center of your chest.
- Now, become aware of a gift that is gracing your life in this moment. Perhaps, it is simply being alive and aware, here and now. Perhaps, it is someone or something that you love or care about. Perhaps, it is a love for Source, for that which is beyond understanding.
- Allow yourself to feel these feelings of gratitude, love and caring as you continue to breathe in and out through the center of your chest.
- Now take a deep breath in through the center of your chest and hold it for a moment. As you release your breath, feel these feelings radiating throughout your entire body.
- Feel the aliveness, love, caring, gratitude in every atom, and every cell of your body.
- Feel the vibrancy of your inner energy body.
- When you are ready gently open your eyes.

(Note: You can record this meditation in your own voice and play it as you relax until you can automatically enter this state. You can also find this and other meditations to download at www.laskow.net.)

To underscore the power of the Conscious Heart Focus, I received a letter from a woman who had done the practice in one of my Holoenergetic seminars. She and her husband both were HIV positive. In the letter, she shared that she had intended to take her own life after the seminar in what would be the last volitional act of her life. However, when the seminar ended she felt that "a huge weight has been lifted from my spirit. My experience today has granted me a vision of hope and peace." That night after the seminar, she went home and conceived a baby with her husband. Thanks to tuning into her own heart, she conceived new life instead of ending her own. Nine months later the child was born HIV negative and has remained so.

Given such a profound transformational healing, imagine what evoking the loving presence and the power of forgiveness can do in your life.

Before we do the Holoenergetic Forgiveness Process, and before we further practice the Presence that creates the space for forgiveness to occur, let's consider one more obstacle to forgiveness — our perception of reality.

FOR GIVING
LOVE

CHAPTER 3

HOW REAL IS REALITY?

The transpersonal self that transcends personal boundaries remains as the experiencer or distinct from what's experienced. The transpersonal self may first come into awareness with the awakening of the inner witness or observer of experience that remains distinct from the contents of consciousness such as thoughts, feelings, sensations or images.
— *Frances Vaughan*

Love and truth have no opposite. The "opposite" of love is the appearance of separation, which doesn't exist, so love has no opposite. The "opposite" of truth is falsehood, which doesn't exist, it only appears to, so truth has no opposite.
— *Leonard Laskow*

We've all heard the saying, "Seeing is believing." But, it might be truer yet that "believing is seeing." We tend to rely on our five physical senses to guide us through the world. At the same time, we filter these signals through the invisible filters of feelings, thoughts, beliefs, programming, and conditioning.

Our Senses: Windows on the World or Projection Booths?

In their book Beyond Biofeedback, Elmer and Alyce Green point out that when we say, "My finger hurts," it might be more accurate to say, "Agitation of free nerve endings in my finger are being projected onto brain areas that, when activated, and when attention is properly focused therein, give a feeling of pain." This is what we mean by "body consciousness" or "sense perception." In the process of interpreting information from our senses, we give our own meaning to the messages coming into our minds from all our sense organs. We filter all the sensory information through our past experiences and beliefs. What comes out the other side of these filters are our present perceptions colored by our past conditioning.

Let's take for example something we often do casually without much consideration. We put our feet up on a table or desk or we sit cross-legged. In some cultures, however, showing the bottoms of one's feet is an outrageous insult. The same action that would get no response in Italy would cause a riot in Iran.

We filter sensory information through our past experiences and beliefs.

Even more importantly, the beliefs we hold within us tend to become self-fulfilling prophecies, reinforced by the external world. We select from the vast possibilities of outer experiences and interpretations that support our inner perceptions. We may not even be seeing what we are actually looking at in the moment. Let's say you take the same walk every day and have done so for years. How much of the scenery are you seeing anew? Or, are you simply re-picturing a memory of what you've seen in the past? To take perception a level deeper, you might not even be seeing what you looked at in the past. You might be seeing what you believed you saw in the past! As Anaïs Nin said, "What we see is not what is, it is who we are."

Of course, it would be challenging to reinvent reality every moment of every day. So, it's helpful that our filters become structures in our consciousness and provide us with a semblance of continuity in an infinite and ever-changing reality. Because we generally don't distinguish what we are seeing from the filters we are looking through, we often unconsciously use those filters to project our beliefs, feelings, and structured perceptions onto the external world. It is as if we had an invisible movie projector within our minds. From the projection booth of our consciousness, we are constantly running a movie made up of all our past structured experiences. The filters we used to interpret our sensory messages have now become a film. The plot of that movie has been determined by future anticipation of past experiences!

The "movie" we've made is projected onto the external world so that the new experiences before us are all intermingled with old experiences from our past. We're rarely aware of our projections. Therefore, it is often very difficult to sort the new information we are receiving from the old film we're projecting. To answer that question "Do we create our own reality?" we most definitely create our own experience of reality. And, through the filter of old reality, we quite often do create our new reality — which is much like the old one.

So, in our interactions with the external world, we both filter information coming in and project information from inside us outward. In this way our own "movie" has an effect on the world outside us. We are observer participants, or better yet director / actor / audience behind our own invisible projector. This projector metaphor can help explain why and how our beliefs can and do create our reality.

Energetically, our projections comprise a set of frequencies that, when matched by the object of those projections, can create an enhanced response, actually encouraging into being the quality that is projected. Let's imagine you are an individual who is uncomfortable around strangers. You find yourself in a new setting, and subconsciously your facial expression and body language projects protection and guardedness. Would it be far-fetched to imagine that the individuals you encounter subconsciously reflect back to you the guardedness they see in your own face?

In this way a projection can become self-fulfilling. That's why lovers seem to have such a glow. They are basking in the projected adoration that brings their inner beauty to the surface. Similarly, if your projector sees hostility, anger and abuse everywhere, it's not surprising to have those projections fulfilled as well.

The filters structured in consciousness are at work even in the seemingly simple perception of sensations. For example, in my seminars, I sometimes have people put one hand in a bucket of hot water and the other in a bucket of ice-cold water. They leave their hands there for about fifteen seconds and then take them out and put them both simultaneously into a bucket of tepid water between the outer buckets. Then, I ask the participants to describe what they feel in each hand. They report that the hand that has been in the ice water senses the tepid water as warm; the hand that has been in the hot water senses the tepid water as cool.

On One Hand, the Water Feels Cool and on the Other Hand …

How can the very same bucket of water seem warm to one hand and cool to the other? From the perspective of the sensing hands — that is, the body consciousness — this is a dualistic paradox. Just as Einstein said that a problem cannot be solved at the level it was created, this sensory paradox cannot be resolved at the level of the buckets, or the linear mind. When confronted with this vexing paradox, the mind does what it knows how to do. It decides. It chooses either / or. From the limited perspective of the linear mind, the bucket temperature cannot be hot and cold simultaneously.

However, there is another part of us, the observer self which I call the Aware Witness that has a broader and more integrative awareness. The Aware Witness is aware of the sensations and also knows where the hands have been just moments before. To the Aware Witness, the senses are only part of the informational input. It perceives the whole process, including the previous conditioning that informs the present perception. This observer part of our self can rise above the "dueling dualities" perceived by our senses, and is able to see the bigger picture.

If you were to do the bucket experiment for yourself, you probably wouldn't be upset at the water seeming both warm and cool at the same time. You would be aware of how the previous conditioning of putting your hands in hot and cold water was influencing your present perception. Your Aware Witness would tell you, "Sense perception is only part of the issue here. There is more to be considered." When confronted with the seeming paradox, you would instinctively shift your awareness to a higher level to resolve it.

But... when emotionally charged issues that bring painful feelings into the foreground are activated, this wiser witnessing part of ourselves can no longer be accessed. The "still, small voice" of the Aware Witness is overridden by conditioned feelings. We forget that we are interpreting reality solely on the basis of our sensations and interpretations based on past experiences that are likely to be distorted.

When we get plugged into emotionally charged issues, the Aware Witness is overridden by conditioned feelings.

To better appreciate how we get pulled into these emotional sinkholes and how we might extract ourselves, let's explore the bucket analogy in more detail. Let's say the bucket on the left represents the past, the one on the right is the future, and the bucket in the middle our present reality. The past bucket represents past conditioning, memories, and experiences. Whereas the future bucket represents expectations, anticipation, wishes, desires, and hopes. The middle bucket representing the present is "what's so" now and also the integration of opposites.

Accepting "what is" (middle bucket) rather than perceiving from the distortions of the conditioned personality, beliefs, or expectations, opens a portal to expanded awareness in the moment. Because perceptions in this state of expanded awareness are less distorted, the actions or non-actions resulting from them will be more appropriate.

"What is" can also come in the form of illness or infirmity. Accepting the "is-ness" of the situation, along with any thoughts and feelings (pleasant or unpleasant) that come up, likewise can engender presence. We can call being with what is "acceptance." Acceptance is the space in which "what is" occurs. Most often the "what is" that is occurring in the moment is referring to the content, the event taking place. Shifting attention to context is a portal to presence. By consciously shifting attention to the space in which the event occurs — the context — we open this portal.

Acceptance is not to be confused with resignation, which is withdrawal of presence. Staying present with "what is" is the key to transformation and healing. We've often heard the saying, "What you can love, you can heal." When we withdraw or obscure presence through denial, distraction, or simply ignoring a signal, we lose our capacity to transform or heal the situation. By being present with the situation or condition as it is — i.e., unconditioned acceptance — we take the first step toward healing into wholeness through love. In my research, when I unconditionally accepted the existence of the bacteria and the cancer cells, I moved into resonance with their consciousness. While in this field of loving acceptance, I introduced the intention to change their behavior. Their growth rate was then substantially reduced. (See appendix 3: Healer Intention)

While it might seem like a contradiction — to accept what we have, yet still want something else — it really isn't. It's just a subtle distinction that has more to do with attachment than desire. Although you can have a desire for a certain outcome, the key is not to be attached to that outcome. Desire is the fuel that moves us toward a fuller life. Attachment limits the fulfillment of that desire by narrowing the options, insisting that it has to be a certain way. A simple way to want or intend yet not be attached to outcome is to ask and then allow.

To continue with the bucket analogy, let's have the outer buckets represent the subject and the object, and the middle bucket represent "what is" — the tepid temperature. So when we say, "I love you," the bucket on one side is the "I," the bucket on the other is "you" and the middle "what is" bucket is simply "love." In other words, subject and object are positioned perceptions creating the illusion of opposites and the appearance of separation. As with the sensations of hot and cold, subject and object are the content of awareness. But more than content is needed for true contentment! Awareness provides context and meaning. From the higher, deeper and broader view of the witness in tune with the Source, opposites are illusion.

Opposites — An Opposing Point of View

Consider that cold isn't the "opposite" of hot. Cold is merely the relative absence of energy, expressed as temperature. Nor is dark the opposite of light. It is the relative absence of light. In a similar way, electricity is neither positive nor negative. Electrical charge is the absence or presence of electrons. From these physical examples, we might extrapolate to the metaphysical. Evil is not the opposite of good and hell is not the opposite of heaven. Both represent the absence of the realization of Oneness. All opposites and dualities are illusory creations of mind. Likewise, love and truth have no opposite. The "opposite" of love is the appearance of separation, which doesn't exist, so love has no opposite. The opposite of truth is falsehood, which also doesn't exist. It is merely the absence of truth.

As previously noted in the tepid water analogy, one can't resolve the problem at the level at which the problem exists. When we allow ourselves to be present in the space of the moment that both includes and transcends seemingly opposite positions, we find the peace of unity. Integrating opposites into unity also applies to interpretations of the past and projections onto the future.

When we allow ourselves to be present in the space of the moment that both includes and transcends seemingly opposite positions, we find the peace of unity.

As Rumi said back in the thirteenth century, "Out beyond ideas of wrongdoing and right doing, there is a field. I'll meet you there." We can be present with that field whenever we remember: All opposites or dualities are illusory creations of mind.

The opposites that emerge from our limited points of view, from the senses alone and from past experience are "relative" truths. Just as the middle bucket of water feels warm or cold relative to the hand's most recent prior experience, sensory input and past memories cannot encompass the "whole" truth. When we transcend to a level of awareness beyond the buckets — i.e., that the experience of hot or cold is relative to prior experience — we can integrate the opposites that stem from positionality.

When we expand our awareness to recognize that perception is always relative based on past conditioning, we can see beyond both poles to a direct perception of what's so. Awareness of the relativity of truth, at the level of duality, helps us to dis-identify with the content of awareness and our attachment to form. Once we release attachment to content, what remains is the context — awareness itself. This awareness is experienced as inner peace. It reminds us that all separation, all sense of opposites is illusory from this aware perspective.

In her book The Inward Arc, Frances Vaughan comments:

> "Wholeness is based on a balance and integration of opposites, not on getting rid of what we don't like. When we feel an inconsistency or conflict between inner experience and outer expression, between persona and shadow, fear and love, life and death, body and mind, or any other pairs of opposites, we experience pain and tension. According to the ancient Hindu scriptures, the Upanishads, wherever there is other - there is fear, for fear is born of duality. We can be released from fear only when we recognize the unity of opposites and learn to balance the polarities of emotional experience in a context of healing awareness."

Have you noticed how much of our waking consciousness is focused on getting rid of what we don't want? What if, as Frances Vaughan suggests, we expand our circle of acceptance to include even what we don't want? That is what forgiveness is. It is bringing into the circle of acceptance that which we have judged as "unlovable." The energy liberated in letting go of obsolete stories of blame and shame that hold our judgment (especially of ourselves) in place can now be used to bring love and freedom to ourselves and anyone else in our field.

Forgiveness is bringing into the circle of acceptance that which we have judged as "unlovable."

From Dueling Dualities to Dynamic Duo Dance Partners

In the physical domain, seeming opposites usually don't disappear completely. Even the cancer cells I worked with didn't disappear; they just decreased in number. However, we can shift our perspective to a higher level of awareness — from dueling dualities to dynamic duo dance partners. Let's take perhaps the most obvious duality in human existence — feminine and masculine, representing respectively the yin and yang principles. If you are familiar with the yin and yang symbol, it is unlikely you have concluded yin is right and yang is wrong … or yang is right and yin is wrong.

Yet based on our experience and perspective coming from being male or female in this world, we may feel at odds with what we call "the opposite sex." Gender difference is how John Gray's book Men Are from Mars, Women Are from Venus became a bestseller.

Let's use the bucket analogy once again and imagine that all the women put their hands in the hot bucket and all the men put their hands in the cold bucket. Naturally, when the women remove their hands from the hot bucket and put them in the tepid middle bucket, their experience tells them the middle bucket is cool. The men, of course, when they move their hand from the cold bucket to the middle bucket, will insist that bucket is warm. With only their perceptual experience to guide them, both the men and the women will insist their perspective is "right." We know that what they are reporting is relative truth, based on past conditioning.

In reality, neither is right or wrong. But you can imagine that when all women agree that the water is cool and all men agree that the water is warm, there is a natural disagreement based on the previous conditioning of their respective water temperature. For women, the conditioning, in part, is represented biologically and physiologically by their genetic makeup, hormones, and conditioning associated with their gender. And of course the same is true for men. The reality of "what is," is influenced by their conditioning and physiology. We can see many different applications of this in politics, nationalism, and religion.

Like the legendary blind men describing the elephant, each one insists the elephant is their experience of it. For the man touching the trunk, the elephant is long and thin. For the one wrapped around its leg, an elephant is tall and pillar shaped. The one hugging its girth insists it is large and thick. And so on.

The bucket experiment reveals the illusory reality we live in. As we will see later, the process of forgiveness can help us to transcend relative reality while we are still here. Forgiveness helps us to shine a light for others to do the same. That light we are shining is neither a particle nor a wave, but it has the potential to express both. It's not surprising that Jesus was symbolically born of the unitive asexual virgin rather than the male-female duality.

One way to experience the shift into the "neutral" of the middle bucket — into present awareness — is to breathe in and out slowly through the center of your chest and recall feelings of love or joy, happiness. (See the Conscious Heart Focus exercise in the previous chapter.) These expansive heartfelt feelings are a portal to presence, to unitive awareness. Unitive awareness inherently transcends the appearance of opposites; it inherently integrates polarities and dualities.

When we have the experience of integrating opposites, we naturally and automatically release identification with polarizing perspectives. As relative content is neutralized, the significance of shared context expands. When we are with our experience alone — as in having a hand in one or the other outer buckets — we experience reality as an either / or situation. We insist that the middle bucket is warm or cool, based on past recent experience, and it seems absurd and impossible that it can be both at once.

Why is this important?

The conditioned automatic mind must use defense mechanisms to defend its interpretation of reality and destroy other alternatives. The conditioned mind will seek to deny, to reject, to suppress, to judge, to condemn, to disown, or to project. It will fervently insist that either the right hand or the left hand is right or wrong. When we are not conscious of the unitive presence, we live as if the neutral, tepid water bucket is either warm or cold all the time, when in fact, it's neither warm nor cold.

The wound, the suffering we so often experience and imagine is

the "stuff" of life is, in reality, a result of living in the either / or
reality based on our sensory perceptions coupled with our disowned
shadow past that has not been integrated into the unity. When we
allow forgiveness to lift us out of judging past situations and circumstances (and unconsciously projecting those onto the future), we
experience the both / and level of awareness where no problem exists. Both / and expresses unity, while either / or represents duality.

The acceptance that comes with forgiveness is not denial, which
is the disconnection from presence. Acceptance is being so fully present that the past perceived problem is absorbed by Unity. That's why
the Conscious Heart Focus process is such a valuable tool. It opens
the heart portal in preparation for forgiveness, love, and freedom.

---

*Acceptance is being so fully present that the past perceived problem
is absorbed by Unity.*

Focusing on opposites is neither good nor bad, right nor wrong.
Experiencing contrast and differentiation is part of Oneness experiencing Itself. It is an essential part of our human journey — and
necessary in order for us to return "home." Manifestation of form
in the physical world requires differentiation as we saw in the Game
of Awakening.

In the poem, Outwitted, Edwin Markham writes:
He drew a circle that shut me out-
Heretic, rebel, a thing to flout.
But love and I had the wit to win:
We drew a circle and took him in!

In a similar way love "overgrows" duality, making a circle that is
all-encompassing.

In the next chapter, we go deeper into "loving presence" and the process of Holoenergetic Healing so that regardless of external circumstances, polarities, and seeming separation, we can always establish ourselves in the field of wholeness, oneness and love.

For now, here is a simple, foundational way to practice presence and align with the unitive field. The Grounding, Aligning and Centering Breath is an excellent practice for learning to match breath, energy, and visualization to tune ourselves up to start the day, create peaceful presence before significant meetings or negotiations, or to remind ourselves of what the "real" reality is, regardless of circumstances.

THE GROUNDING, ALIGNING, AND CENTERING BREATH

These three simple steps will have you in a state of peaceful presence within minutes.

Grounding:

Begin by taking several slow, deep breaths. Then, as you breathe in, imagine that you are drawing in energy from the core of the earth up through the base of your spine to your heart. As you gently exhale your breath, imagine the energy being released into the center of your chest, into your heart center grounding you to the earth.

Aligning:

In your relaxed and grounded state, imagine above your head a radiant sun, your transpersonal or soul space. Sense or imagine that you are drawing your next breath in from this radiant sun down through the top of your head and release your breath into your heart center. You have now aligned with your spiritual nature.

Centering:

With your next breath, sense or imagine simultaneously drawing energy up from the core of the earth and down from this radiant sphere through the top of your head. Release your breath into your heart center, fusing the energy coming from above and below — fusing spirit and matter, the masculine and feminine, heaven and earth, resolving duality into unity in your heart.

Now you are grounded, aligned, and centered. This process alters your state of consciousness, allowing you to maintain an aware presence and access information through the intuitive heart and mind. As a breathing meditation, you can simply continue to breathe in and out through your heart center, or follow with the Conscious Heart Focus.

(Note: You can record this meditation in your own voice and play it back until you can automatically put yourself in this state.

You can also find this and other meditations to download at www. laskow.net.)

CHAPTER 4

HOLOENERGETIC HEALING

The greatest source of our suffering stems from the illusion that we
are only our body and mind.
— Leonard Laskow

Love is Oneness in action.
— Nisargadatta

Healing ultimately takes place on a level we can only call grace, cou-
pled with willingness on our part.
— Leonard Laskow

"Your work is to heal with love."

That was the initial revelation I received nearly forty years ago, and that impulse has guided my work ever since. The technical name I've given the work I do is "Holoenergetic Healing," and the Holoenergetic Forgiveness Process is a portal to both healing and love. So, what is healing? And what is love?

The original meaning of the word healing is "to restore whole-ness" or "to make whole." When we "remember" we bring together the dismembered, fragmented, or unacknowledged parts of our-selves, and the larger picture reveals itself. In a civilization where only matter matters (i.e., where only the physical, measurable world of form is considered real) achieving both manifest and unmanifest wholeness is particularly challenging.

Like most of my contemporaries growing up in middle class America in the 1940s and 1950s, my early days had been consciously and unconsciously structured as a means to an end. I had learned to focus on future goals — like becoming a doctor — and was con-ditioned both by past experiences as well as abiding beliefs. I was oblivious to the fragrance of the moment. I was unaware of how my beliefs and conditioning had refracted and filtered the light of pure awareness into the personal "me" of conditioned desire and aversion.

The epiphany I had while meditating revealed to me that my mis-sion was to heal with love. This revelation was quite a blessing. For a number of years after that I focused on healing with love, the title of my first book. Subsequently, I came to realize that the deeper work was to heal into wholeness with love.

So what is the relationship between love and healing? What is love and how does it help us to access wholeness?

As a functional definition, love is the awareness of relatedness and the impulse toward unity.

Love is the awareness of relatedness and the impulse toward unity.

When you focus on what it is you want to change, first acknowl-edging your relationship to it and then coming into loving acceptance of the issue, you have gone a long way toward revealing wholeness. On the other hand, if you deny, disown, or dismiss the situation that requires healing, you've created separation, which veils and obscures wholeness. As was said before: What you can love, you can heal.

Now of course there are many other ways to change something. You can cut it with a knife, you can hit it with a hammer, you can use some other form of physical force or leverage. Or you can shift from trying to fix, move, or rearrange the discrete particles of life and directly impact the field through love.

Love is the universal harmonic. Just like a magnetic field magnetizes individual pieces of iron into a coherent configuration, using the harmonizing power of love is a more subtle yet far more efficient way of making change. When you change the field template, you change what the field manifests physically as form.

A coherent loving field by itself, even without any specific intention, is enough to stimulate healing because this essence of love — being one with everything — is resonant with wholeness. As you experience coherent loving energy, you begin to vibrate at the frequency of the universal harmonic. The separating dissonances begin to fade, and you are reminded of your essential nature. Similarly, the goal of healing is to come into coherent resonance with and to ultimately merge with your essential nature, which is synonymous with wholeness.

It follows that a Holoenergetic practitioner's greatest gift is to be so fully present that their client's essential nature, which is one with the practitioner's, is resonantly activated. Ideally, this shared field of undistorted, nonjudgmental awareness or witnessing then becomes the context in which all subsequent therapeutic interaction transpires. Since "problems" for which clients seek help ultimately derive from the illusion of separation from one's essential nature, true healing can only occur in this contextual field of wholeness, which simultaneously includes and transcends all phenomena.

Is Illness a Symptom of Separation?

Illness is frequently associated with a sense of separation of one part of our self from another, of our self from others and our environment, and from our own connection with our essential nature. Truly, it's not possible for us to actually be separated from our Aware Witness and wholeness. If we are part of wholeness, how can we be separate from it? We may have the perception of separation, which certainly "feels" real but is a perceptional illusion. Because this appearance of separation resists the underlying reality of wholeness, it must take energy to maintain this illusion. In fact, it takes an enormous amount of energy to keep wounds suppressed, buried, and disowned. It likewise requires energy to construct and maintain the stories that cast blame on ourselves and others.

Using energy to sustain the illusion of separation means that energy is not available for other things, such as maintaining health and fulfilling our dreams. If we can release the energy of separation by bringing ourselves back into wholeness, into awareness of our essential nature, that energy becomes available to support natural healing. The body knows how to heal itself. When we release the energy of separation through love and forgiveness, we transform what is held separate into unity. This energy of love facilitates the healing process.

There are times when just that release through love is sufficient for healing — physical healing, emotional healing, and mental healing. Furthermore, we can heal even as we experience unhappy and unloving emotions. Even when people are angry and full of hate, physical healing can still take place because the body knows how to heal. As a simple example, if you cut your finger — even if you are upset with yourself about it — your body will naturally begin to heal the cut.

In spiritual healing, however, love is both sufficient and necessary.

The Holoenergetic Healing process — through Holoenergetic Tracing — helps you trace an issue back to its experiential root in a way that you deeply experience the separating incident. The separation may have occurred in your mother's womb or in early childhood. It could have been an actual event that happened, a misperception, or a misinterpretation that got crystalized as a belief. As long as you can directly re-experience the experience, you can bring to it the heat of emotions experienced through the light of awareness. Then, you can change the emotional charge associated with the situation. Releasing the emotional charge frees you from the conditioning of the past.

Holoenergetic Healing is healing using the energy of the whole that is greater than the sum of the parts. Remember, it takes energy to maintain separation. Ultimately, there is no separation other than what the mind creates and the emotions maintain. As we release the appearance of separation and bring ourselves into wholeness, a tremendous amount of energy is liberated. The simple work of healing is to release the illusion of separation and to allow deep wholeness to emerge. To the extent that we align ourselves with wholeness that we disconnected from, deep healing has occurred.

The simple work of healing is to release the illusion of separation and to allow wholeness to emerge.

Holoenergetic Healing occurs on all levels, including the physical, emotional, mental, and spiritual aspects of our being. For those who are seeking physical healing, the process is effective. Not in every case, of course. Just as is true with allopathic medicine, homeopathy, or any other form of healing, there are many variables involved. Regarding physical healing, my research with bacteria and tumor cells indicates that by holding an image and/or thought with clear intention within a coherent field of love, we can affect nonhuman living systems as well. My research suggests a strong role of consciousness in healing.

How Holoforms Can Impact Whole Forms

Holoforms are energetic patterns that exist in the energy fields interpenetrating and surrounding the body. These patterns can induce illness in the physical body. While we may not be able to "see" them, we can energetically detect them and recognize when and where they are operating. These holoforms usually originate in choices and interpretations we make about our experiences, often at an early age. Although those interpretations are no longer valid and may well have been distorted at the time, we continue to hold them as structures in consciousness, where they shape our present experience and perpetuate the illusion of separation.

Not only does a holoform influence how we receive experience and how we express ourselves, it also acts like an energetic template that directs and configures the molecular, atomic, and subatomic activity of the body. In the case of a dysfunctional pattern, a holoform may give rise to illness.

By focusing attention on a thought, feeling, sensation, or belief associated with the old pattern, we can recreate the entire holoform. That's why I call the pattern a holoform. As with a hologram, the whole is contained in each of its parts. Holoenergetic Healing allows us to go back to the source of the dysfunctional pattern — the moment in which we chose to interpret a particular event in a certain way — to take responsibility for our choice and to choose again.

A key part of choosing again is recognizing the three levels of healing and recognizing which level or levels you are ready, willing, and able to experience.

The Three T's of Change

Holoenergetic Healing can take place on three levels — Translation, Transformation, and Transcendence. People often ask how Holoenergetic Healing is different from other forms of healing that work at an energetic level — like acupuncture or homeopathy. The differences have to do with these three levels of change.

The first level of change is shifting energy from one place in the body to another place where it's more useful for healing. This shift is called **translation.**

On the second level, the healer can **transform** the energy by bringing the person being healed closer to wholeness, closer to their essential nature, thus changing the way the energy is structured in consciousness. Such transformative change releases the energy that's bound up in separation.

The third level of healing **transcends** the old energy pattern completely by shifting to an entirely new way of perceiving and experiencing reality.

Acupuncture, homeopathy, bodywork, and allopathic medicine are all good examples of translational change where healing is facilitated by shifting and balancing the energies. Holoenergetic Healing is an example of transformational change. By releasing and reforming the pattern that underlies an illness, we release tremendous reserves of life-force energy that can transform an individual's entire life. When Holoenergetic Healing is taken to its highest level, there are those who, in the course of healing, come to transcend identification with body and mind. For those people, events at the level of personality no longer matter as they once did. This is what I call Opening to Oneness.

In Holoenergetic Healing, change occurs through awareness, love, and conscious choice. Change is first generated on the emotional, mental, intellectual, and spiritual levels and then on the physical level. Translation, transformation, and transcendence are three ways to release and reform energetically. Each is associated with a change in conscious awareness. Let's look at each of the "3 T's of Change" in more detail.

In Holoenergetic Healing, change occurs through awareness, love and conscious choice.

Translation

When a skilled linguist translates a thought or feeling from one language to another, the form changes but the substance of the message changes little, if at all. Thus, a love poem would convey approximately the same sentiments in English as it would in French, Chinese, or Russian. Similarly, in Holoenergetic Healing a translation of energy changes the core issue little, if at all, while it does change the "language" in which the Holoenergetic pattern is expressed.

For example, when a man goes out for a long run to work out anger toward his boss, he's translating his angry feelings into action. However, the core issue that produced his anger hasn't changed. What has changed is that the man has translated that same energy from the language of thoughts and feelings to the language of physical movement. He has found a way to use his angry energy to gain the benefit of exercise and release.

Translation occurs on an emotional level when you shift an emotion to a location where it can be dissipated, such as when you translate anger into action or shift one emotion or feeling to another. Contracted feelings such as pity can be translated into empathy. Stubbornness can be translated into persistence. Judgmental attitudes can be translated into discernment. Negative beliefs, such as "I am not worthy of love," can be translated into affirmations, such as "I am lovable."

The key idea to keep in mind with translational change is that the core issue doesn't resolve; that is, the underlying Holoenergetic pattern that triggered the circumstance remains intact and continues to affect you. The pattern will continue to function as a dis-harmonious energy, reproducing and attracting the unwanted thoughts, feelings, or actions until you access and transform the core issue itself.

Translation can work well on a symptomatic level and is an important part of the healing process. Imagery and visualization can be valuable in dissipating symptoms and can even result in a cure. In practice, a symptom is translated, or converted, into a symbol or image. When the image is changed, frequently the symptom changes as well.

For example, herpes can be treated symptomatically on a translational level. The lesion, often experienced as a burning sensation, can be visualized symbolically as a red-hot burning ember. Imagining cold water poured over the hot ember symbolically extinguishes it. When on a physical level, the redness, pain, and swelling disappeared, translational change has occurred.

In acupuncture, and with some body therapies, the practitioner may shift energy flow from one area of the body to another to bring balance or shift the energy to a place where it's more useful.

Changing the perception that the glass is half empty to the perception that the glass is half full is an example of translational change since the amount of water (the level of conscious awareness) in the glass remains the same. This change in perception can initiate an epigenetic placebo effect, a change outside the genes and the body. The way you relate to a memory, for example, can actually influence the way your genes manufacture proteins that impact your health and well-being. You are probably already familiar with the placebo effect, where taking a sugar pill and believing it is a pharmacological drug can actually change your physiology as if you had taken the drug. While this may seem quite extraordinary, it still represents translational change. The symptom is miraculously alleviated, while the underlying condition remains unchanged.

Usually, translation precedes transformation. When you translate a symptom to an image or simple statement, you can directly address the critical incident, choices, and core beliefs. You can then finally uncover the positive life-force energies, and the transformational process can begin. By releasing and reforming, blending and evolving the image, you complete the Holoenergetic transformation.

Transformation

Transformation requires a deeper level of consciousness wherein you are aware not only of the discomfort of the present circumstances you want to change, but also of the source or underlying Holoenergetic pattern that generates and maintains those circumstances. By accessing the source of an illness, emotion, or belief — the identification with mind structures — you expand your awareness. When awareness of the source of the illness is coupled with consciously evoked energy changes, Holoenergetic Healing occurs. This Holoenergetic Healing process is more than a translation of energy from one domain to another. It involves insightful psychological understanding along with energetic release. Together, these transform unwarranted patterns of energy in the form of feelings and thoughts, choices and decisions, beliefs and attitudes associated with illness.

With translational change, awareness expands and contracts continuously within any given level of consciousness. One moment, you might be aware of only the page you are reading; at the next, you become aware of the room around you. When you are sleepy you are less aware; when you are alert you are more aware. Holoenergetic change takes place when your access to awareness expands in an enduring way through a shift to a higher level of consciousness or awakening. As Ralph Metzner says in Opening to Inner Light, transformation requires that "the structure and functioning of our psyche become different."

Holoenergetic change takes place when your access to awareness expands in an enduring way through a shift to a higher level of consciousness.

_Each level of consciousness has its own pattern of vibration, structure, and function. The vibrational qualities at higher levels of consciousness expand and reshape the content of your awareness, changing your perceptions, thoughts, feelings, choices, and beliefs.

Transformation involves moving toward a new level of consciousness wherein there is a greater awareness and ability to see the truth about yourself. The energetic patterns that produce illness are like anchors holding a given structure or pattern in consciousness. When those patterns are released, you are freed to rise to a higher level of consciousness and, thus, to a greater awareness of the source of the illness. At higher vibrational levels, you are able to gain access to consciousness that lies at the source and dictates the form taken by an energy pattern.

Transformational healing can occur on physical, emotional, mental, or spiritual levels, and the results can be expressed in any and all of these levels.

At a physical level, transformation is frequently, but not always, reflected as a change in behavior and appearance. For example, the Bible recounts that Saul, after his transformational experience, changed from an enemy to a defender of the faith. Similarly, criminals who've experienced transformational healing epiphanies have been known to become exemplary citizens. Still others, after transformational experiences, find themselves confirmed in their spiritual practices and life paths with no obvious outward changes. As the Zen masters have said, "Before enlightenment, chop wood and carry water. After enlightenment, chop wood and carry water."

As Metzner notes in Opening to Inner Light, "Bodily appearance may or may not be altered when consciousness and self are transformed ... in illness and healing recovery, a physical form and appearance may change drastically. Anyone who has undergone the 'remission' of a malignant tumor, spontaneously or as a result of psychic healing, has brought about a kind of a chemical transformation of the physical elements of the body."

At the emotional level, transformational change brings lasting awareness and integration of expansive and contracted feelings as well as an awareness of their origin. You can translate feelings of

stress to feelings of relaxation through certain breathing exercises
... and, you can transform those feelings when you take breathing
techniques a step further using them to connect with the source of
our stress.

At the mental level, transformational change allows you to assume responsibility for reacting to the original traumatic experience, given the consciousness available to you at that time. You then
release or evolve the unwanted energy form it produces and then
make a new choice for change. You are empowered to restructure
your psyche to support these harmonious beliefs so you can make
entirely new choices, free of imprisoning illusions. You gain the ability to hear the body's whispers instead of waiting for the shout of
illness or trauma.

At the spiritual level, the enhanced awareness associated with
the transformational process is often expressed as a greater sense
of self and recognition of trans-personal values such as joy and
gratitude as well as the experience of synchronicity and serendipity.
The more aware you are, the more correlations you make, and the
more things you can relate to others and yourself. With expanded
awareness, you gain self-knowledge and understanding. With greater understanding, there comes more forgiveness and compassion,
less judgment and blame. When you live your understanding and
compassion, it becomes wisdom. Wisdom is the compassionate understanding of truth.

Wisdom is the compassionate understanding of truth

Above all and underneath all, there is the power of love — the
awareness of relatedness and the impulse toward unity. Love and
the wholeness it reveals facilitates your ability to relate, link, and
connect. When you relate to what is so, love brings you to truth.

Love allows you to relate your illness to its origin and a greater sense of yourself as a co-creator of your reality. Your love can also transform every emotion and every thought by relating it to its origin. Your love is the most powerful of all transforming energies.

We can transform and grow through love and joy or through pain and suffering. Certainly, pain and suffering have helped many to become more aware of the origin of the difficulty. But let's remember that we can also become aware through love and joy. With love and joy, come forgiveness and the ability to stop judging and blaming ourselves and others. We can let go of our defenses and see the truth of what is. The love and joy of transformation become guiding principles, giving us the directions we need to make that choice for growth.

When you transform a situation in your life, you gain access to energy that you've been using to maintain your separation from yourself and others. When you maintain the illusion of separation, with its limiting beliefs, it is as if you are putting all of your strength and weight to push against a door — and behind that door is a vast amount of vital, usable energy. When you let go of the illusion of separation, through transformation and transcendence, the door suddenly bursts open. You now have available to you all the radiant energy that was trapped behind that door plus all the energy you were using to hold the door shut.

When we transform a situation in our lives, we gain access to energy that we've been using to maintain our separation from ourselves and others.

To use again the analogy of the half-full glass, through transformation the glass becomes filled — sometimes to overflowing as our conscious awareness expands. This is not only a perceptual shift; it

also represents the transformational release of abundant energy —
energy to heal, to grow, to create with.

Transcendence

Transcending can be literally "trance ending" as we experience a
shift in consciousness where we truly see and experience beyond the
veils of separation. We go beyond form to essence, so we transcend
the form that we recently transformed. By initially resonating with
the form, then attuning to its essence, we make a quantum leap, ex-
panding beyond the duality. Now, through essence, we have access
not only to the energy we were using to hold the illusion in place
— we have access to all possible forms of energy because we are
accessing energy beyond form.

Survivors of near-death experiences often report moments of
transcendence. This is understandable because they have not just
transformed form. They have, for that brief moment, transcended
form into essence. Transformation and transcendence both involve
a death of the old form. In transformation, a new and more evolved
form is generated, which is capable of releasing or absorbing more
energy. In transcendence, consciousness leaps beyond the world of
form. We are liberated from form, free to choose and free to be, and
then to re-embrace the form without being identified with or attached to it.

Transformation is a natural part of our evolution, and we are
all capable of transcendence. By consciously choosing to grow toward wholeness, we can experience healing in its fullest sense. This
heightened awareness of our essential nature and wholeness is what
distinguishes healing from cure, which is the resolution of pathol-
ogy. Healing in this transcendent sense goes way beyond physical
cure. Those who have worked in hospice know that when a patient
fully accepts his or her imminent departure from the world of form,
there is a transcendent peace that makes any physical condition ir-
relevant.

With transcendence, our glass is not only filled, but we tap into
the ocean that is the Source of all.

THE 3 T'S AT A GLANCE

Translation changes one form of energy into another without addressing the fundamental issue or cause. For example, we can translate anger into action, stubbornness into persistence, judgment into discernment. However, the core issue doesn't get resolved and continues manifesting the disharmonious energy pattern.

Bottom line: Translation can relieve, reduce or transfer symptoms, yet the causes remain unaddressed.

Transformation accesses the origin of the pattern. Through expanded insight and energetic release, you experience new levels of awareness. By getting to the fundamental cause, you release the energy that has held the pattern in place, making that energy available for positive and proactive manifestation.

Bottom line: Transformation generally involves physical and behavioral changes. Stress transforms to peace and relaxation. You become more responsible for the choices you make. You become more attuned to physical and emotional signals. You may experience greater love, joy, and gratitude.

Transcendence lifts us above any condition and penetrates the veils of separation. We are liberated from the form we seek to change. We become freer to "re-form" the forms in our lives based on newer, deeper and more accurate "in-form-ation."

Bottom line: Transcendence is "trance-ending," as it breaks the trance of separation and allows us to abide as our essential nature.

The Four R's

While change and healing take place on three levels, there is a four-step process to Holoenergetic Healing. Those steps (which we call the four R's) are: Recognize, Resonate, Release and Reform.

Recognize

The first step is to recognize what you want to change. What is the form that's not serving you now? What information do you need now in order to change? There are two levels at which we access this information. The first is the rational, cognitive level — the information you get when you ask the following questions:

- What is the issue or problem I want to focus on?
- What is prompting me to change now?
- How do I see myself contributing to the present circumstances?
- What does this illness or situation keep me from doing, being, or having?
- What does it allow me to do, be, or have?
- What result, outcome, and inner experience do I really want to have?

The second level of **recognize** is intuitive and energetic. Drawing on the non-rational, intuitive aspects of the mind can help us to rediscover the source of limiting patterns...the times in life when we unconsciously made significant decisions that influenced or blocked our subsequent health and well-being.

Resonate

Having recognized the problem, the next stage is called resonate. By focusing your attention on the negative sensation, thought, feeling, or symptom, you come into resonance with it—that is, your awareness begins to vibrate at its frequency. Each holoform has its own unique, natural vibratory frequency. When you come into resonance with this frequency, you become one with the form. Then you can trace it back to its roots. You may need to re-experience the initial or related event completely, especially through following the feelings associated with it.

For example, if you're dealing with a painful incident, you may have to go into the pain to re-experience it rather than intellectually dismissing, disowning, or denying it. If you resonate deeply enough, you will come to understand what it was you really wanted to experience and feel at the time the pain originated. During this resonant phase of the Holoenergetic Tracing Process, people generally get in deeper touch with their pain. While "inside" the pain, they discover what beneficial life-force energies have been thwarted and distorted by the painful core issue. When these life-force energies are unblocked, you can freely feel the calling of the soul.

Some of these life-force energies include:

Security and safety
Vitality and aliveness
Creativity and pleasure
Manifesting successfully
Making a difference in the world
Self-empowerment and self-expression
A sense of belonging, love, and relatedness
Joy and abundance
Knowing who you are, your soul's desire, and mission
Being who you are
Peace and freedom
Unity

Most people, when they penetrate to the essence of a traumatic event or an illness, find that what their soul wanted to express and to experience was one or more of these vital inner experiences: freedom, love, peace, joy, a sense of their own empowerment and creativity, or a feeling of security. For example, they may have received abuse and abandonment, but what they really wanted was love. As Jean Shinoda Bolen has said, "We all come into the world as children who want love, and if we can't get love, we settle for power." Perhaps this sheds light on how perpetrations get perpetuated from one generation to the next.

Release

Finally, to complete the healing, you need to release the old form energetically and replace it with what you really wanted. To release the painful form, you take a deep breath and hold your breath while you're feeling the form intensely. Then, intending to totally and completely dissipate the form, release your breath through the area of the body where you're holding the pattern. Usually, this is the place where the symptom, trauma, or tension manifests itself physically. If you're working with a Holoenergetic practitioner, they will at the same time withdraw the energy from the area using their breath. The release process is like deflating a balloon while somebody else is helping you to collapse it.

Forgiveness is what I call the final release, which is why I treat it separately from the Holoenergetic Healing Process. When the tracing process is complete, whatever is left to forgive becomes apparent.

Reform

Having dissipated the original pattern, you've created a void. Within the void, you can reform (re-form) what is really wanted — peace, love, freedom, empowerment, creativity, security, joy — in the form of a symbol or image that represents the missing inner experience for you.

To summarize, these are the four stages of the Holoenergetic healing process:

- Recognize the issue you want to change.
- Resonate with it.
- Release the form that no longer serves.
- Reform a new form in alignment with what you really want to experience, in alignment with your soul.

THIS IS A SUMMARY OF THE HOLOENERGETIC TRACING PROCESS

Step 1: Recognition

Close your eyes, breathe deeply, and focus your attention on the symptom, issue, or situation you want to change — focus on the problem so that you resonantly connect with it.

Keeping this issue or situation in mind, allow yourself to notice where in your body your awareness is drawn. Focus your attention on that area and become aware of any sensations there, such as pressure, tension, tingling, throbbing.

Example: With a migraine headache, the attention might be

drawn to a throbbing spot behind the temple.

Give that sensation or focus of attention a shape, such as a bright red ball — or any other form that works for you. We will call this the original form.

Step 2: Resonance

In this step we follow the feeling to enhance energetic resonance with what we want to change.

Draw a deep breath in through the form, up into your head, and release your breath from your head back into the form, following your breath with your mind so that you find yourself inside the form. As you penetrate this form with your mind, deep emotions are likely to come up. Allow yourself to feel these emotions... and to travel back mentally to an earlier time when you had similar feelings. Begin to explore the beliefs and emotional patterns you formed around this issue.

Delve even more deeply inside to discover the positive value of this pattern. This might include messages or warnings the pattern has for you... the security or protection it provided... other legitimate needs that you would now like to meet in healthier ways. Intuitively allow this positive life-force energy to assume a symbolic form or image, such as a sun, rose, waterfall, or spiritual figure.

Step 3: Release

This step uses breath, intention, imagery, and energy to release the undesirable pattern.

Until now in this process, you have been imagining yourself inside the form of your troublesome issue or physical symptom. Now, it is time to withdraw your mind from inside the form — but keep in your mind's eye both the new image of your positive life-force energy and the original form.

Release the original dysfunctional form by taking a deep breath and expelling it forcefully — and with it, your picture of the symptom (that bright red ball). Imagine the original form bursting and dissolving like a bubble in water or completely dissipating. At the same time, move your hands as if to forcefully extract the energy from that area of your body. Inhale and expel one more clearing breath. Experience the feeling of freedom from your old pattern.

Step 4: Reformation

By releasing the old form, you have created a void, which you can fill with positive life-force energy during this step.

Focus your attention on the new healing image you created for your positive life-force energy in step 2. Visualize that area of your body that has been giving you trouble and draw the healing image into it with your next indwelling breath. You may also wish to fill the area with the image of healthy-looking organs or tissue... or new, healthy beliefs about yourself. These life-force energies and healing image represent what your soul — that which is simultaneously aware of your uniqueness and unity — wants to experience and express through you.

Complete the healing process by experiencing the Unconditional Love Process. Become aware of a sense of pure, nonjudgmental, boundless love for every aspect of your being. Feel this love as light radiating from your heart, filling your whole body (and flowing out the top of your head like a rainbow fountain). Know that loving presence is your essential nature.

A Holoenergetic Healing Story

A number of years ago, a patient came to me complaining of severe, debilitating low-back pain. The pain was so severe that she had to crawl from her bed to the bathroom in the morning. A CAT scan indicated that she had a ruptured, herniated disk, and her neurosurgeon had scheduled her for a lumbar laminectomy and spinal fusion. That's an operation in which the protruding portion of the ruptured disk is removed and the lumbar vertebrae are fused. She came to me with the hope that she could avoid surgery and also to better understand the meaning of her illness.

As she responded to my questions in the **recognition** phase, she realized that she had a "back-breaking" job, which she performed so perfectly and so responsibly that her boss kept heaping more and more work on her shoulders. As we delved deeper, she got in touch with the shame underlying her perfectionism. She was able to trace the source of her illness back to her relationship with her father, a silent man who withheld his approval and love until she earned it by what she did, not by who she was. Work had become a surrogate father, and her self-esteem now depended on her job, which she felt compelled to do perfectly.

In the **resonance** phase, she was guided to come into resonance with the holoform, the disharmonious energetic pattern, which was located in her lumbar area and consisted of the shame and perfectionism based on her relationship with her father. I had her focus her attention on the Holoenergetic pattern, describe the feelings and images associated with it, and then go back to the earliest time she could recall having similar feelings — a time when she was first developing the belief that she had to be perfect in order to get Daddy's love.

Then, she filled the lumbar area with the healthy image and with a symbolic form that represented what it was she really wanted. In her case, the healthy image was a normal-looking spinal column, without any disk protrusions. Before we started the process, she had an opportunity to study pictures of a healthy spine. At the same time, she had tuned into what she really wanted at the time the pattern formed, which was love.

First, she created a symbolic image representing this love — in her case, an image of her father tucking her in at night and kissing her on the forehead. For other people, love may be represented by such symbols as a sunset, a rose, an animal, an archetypal figure, or the ocean.

After the **release**, she filled the lumbar area with the image of the healthy spine; then she infused it with the image of her loving father. This image represented the positive life-force energy for her — the energy that is aligned with the natural order and harmony of the inherent healing process of the body.

When we fill an area with that positive life-force energy — the energy of her soul — we deeply facilitate the healing process. The infusion of new healthier forms is the **reformation** phase. All her life she had sought this love and acceptance. Now that she had it, she didn't have to seek it outside herself anymore. With reformation came the profoundly healing insight that she could now give herself the love she wanted from others.

During this final reformation phase, I guided her while maintaining an unconditionally loving field with my hands placed in front of her abdomen and over her spine as she was doing the resonance and release work within the field. When she focused her attention on the lumbar area again after release, the pain had disappeared — and it never recurred.

Her neurosurgeon canceled her surgery. Not only was she able to avoid painful surgery and rehabilitation, but upon returning to work, she was promoted to head the international division of a well-known organization and given her own office with a secretary to lighten her workload. She knew that a major transformational shift had occurred in her. She felt self-empowered and was able to give and receive love in a much deeper way.

That's why I call this work transformational. Along with the physical and emotional changes, people's whole lives can change as they release dysfunctional patterns and get in touch with their true nature. To the extent that they can do this, Holoenergetic Healing becomes transcendent.

Now that we understand the levels of Holoenergetic Healing, see the steps, and have experienced Loving Presence and the release of past conditioning, we are ready for the final release — forgiving ourselves.

CHAPTER 5

THE HOLOENERGETIC FORGIVENESS PROCESS

The mystery of life is not a problem to be solved but a reality to be experienced.
— Aart van der Leeuw

The feeling of forgiving ourselves and others is at the heart of our healing work.
— Leonard Laskow

We forgive ourselves and others so we can love without condition.
— Leonard Laskow

Now that we have explored the Holoenergetic Healing Process and have seen how Aware Presence can help us heal, we are ready for the piece d' resistance — or more accurately, the peace d' nonresistance — the Holoenergetic Forgiveness Process. We are now ready to give ourselves unconditioned love and unbounded freedom.

Freedom from what?

Freedom from the attachment to our story and from past conditioning… and not just freedom from, but also freedom to. Freedom to experience love as a constant context rather than a fleeting experience dependent upon circumstance, freedom to fully express our soul's purpose, and freedom to be a beacon for others.

We have said earlier that the suffering in life is about separation from Source — or rather the perception of being separated from Source. In reality, we cannot be separate from Source; we can only forget our connection. The Holoenergetic Forgiveness Process is a way to remember, to reconnect with the disconnected parts in the context of love.

Unconditioned love is not about changing the content of your life, but rather about accessing the ever-present context in which all content arises and subsides. When we realize this, the search for love from the outside ends. Suffering occurs when we identify with the content of love — the people, places, objects, conditions that we associate with our happiness. We free ourselves from suffering when we remember that unconditioned love is the context, the connector of all things. When we experience content through this context, we experience inner peace.

Whenever we make our love about some "thing" (i.e., something manifest on the material plane), we forget that our essential nature is loving awareness. As we said in chapter 2, there is a subtle difference between "unconditioned" love and "non-conditioned" love. Unconditioned love may direct love toward someone or something without condition or attachment to outcome. Non-conditioned love is radiant like the sun and non-directional. Love without condition opens the portal to wholeness.

Both unconditioned and non-conditioned love transcend suffering because they don't identify with anything or anyone as the source of happiness. As such, they are both portals to wholeness. The difference is that non-conditioned love has no object.

All suffering is content. This is also true for hurt, pain, longing; these are all about objects, the content in our lives. The same is true for pleasure. Pleasure can be conditional and fleeting, dependent upon conditions "out there." Beyond pain or pleasure, beyond joy or sadness, when we come home to our essential nature, we find indescribable freedom, peace, and ineffable love.

All suffering is content — or a limited context.

When we practice forgiveness through the Holoenergetic Forgiveness Process, we use this greater context to process the content that is the object of distress. Forgiveness is a tool of the soul because it allows us to manifest simultaneous awareness. Instead of merely noticing the distress, we notice who is doing the noticing.

Releasing the Emotional Charge

The Holoenergetic Forgiveness Process helps us transform the painful situation or memory by releasing the charge we've been holding on to. Practicing the Holoenergetic Forgiveness Process outlined in this chapter will make this field of Oneness more familiar and more easily accessible. In the space of Aware Witness, we become aware of the condition we wish to forgive and release, and we also are aware of what is noticing this.

Being in these two places at once allows us to fully experience all the feelings bundled in the original traumatic event, and at the same time to be in the transcendent space where these feelings of separation from Source are seen to be a misperception of the personality. Holding and feeling the feelings of separation in a field of coherent love is what allows us to discharge the emotionally charged memory. As we experience this sense of One Consciousness, we return to the place we started in the unmanifest and recognize we have been "here" all along.

We forgive ourselves and others so we can love ourselves, others, and life itself without condition. In coming home to our essential nature — unity awareness — we transcend mortality. It is a true portal to Oneness when we are at one with our essential nature, through soul to consciousness itself, and no longer identified with the physical, mental and emotional bodies. This is both transcending and trance ending.

We forgive ourselves and others so we can love ourselves, others, and life itself without condition.

When we experience the content of life through the context of love — as in the Holoenergetic Forgiveness Process — we are simultaneously aware of contrast and unity. In this simultaneous awareness, we experience life through the filter of the soul, not only the personality. While the personality seeks to avoid pain, the soul embraces pain as energy for healing. Here is where we can recognize a subtle difference between "detachment" and "non-attachment." Detachment is contractive; non-attachment is expansive. We detach to separate, to close ourselves off from a painful situation. As children, many of us did that. We experienced a painful trauma and didn't have the resources to deal with it any other way. So we placed the negative experience in "deep storage."

The Holoenergetic Tracing and Holoenergetic Forgiveness Processes help us to safely "re-member" these dismembered parts to liberate them from their "jail cells." In this place of peace and freedom, we can experience the expansive state of non-attachment. With nothing "out there" required to "make us happy," we experience the radiant state of non-attachment. We experience unity by being unity. When we experience our earthly life from this space of non-attachment, we have more freedom and capacity than when we are actively "trying" to detach. Forgiveness helps us to love, to embrace and to accept ourselves. Ultimately, we realize there is no one to forgive because there is only One.

All Forgiveness Is Self-Forgiveness

While it may appear that we are forgiving someone else — or even God or Source — in reality, we forgive ourselves. This realization came to me during a deep meditation many years ago, where I got in touch with what seemed to be a past life. I have no way of knowing if this memory is "real," although the insights gleaned from this experience certainly are.

In this meditation, I had a sense that I was an Essene Master about 3,800 years ago in a Biblical land. I was part of a small group of about a hundred individuals who followed an austere lifestyle based on the prevailing Essene beliefs at that time. At the time, I was about fifty-five years old and I fell in love with one of my followers, a beautiful girl in her early twenties. Although abstinence was one of our practices, in our love for one another, the young woman and I began to have sexual relations in secret. Meanwhile, our group had begun attracting followers from neighboring tribes. This generated concern and envy from other tribal leaders. One night, a rival tribe launched an attack on our group, killing many of our followers, including my loved one.

In deep hurt and despair, I railed at God. "Why did you leave me to live and suffer? For all of my life I've followed your law impeccably. Then, when I opened my heart to love, this is the way that you reward me. If this is the kind of God that you are, I want nothing more to do with you. I reject you."

What I saw in reliving that lifetime from a higher perspective was that God didn't "create" the attack. It was my own judgment of

myself for having broken these laws that I had internally imposed
upon myself and attributed to God. And so it was my own judgment
that brought about the punishment for having breached these laws.
How often is it that our own judgments, consciously or unconsciously, function as resonant attractors that manifest beliefs held within?

Like the rest of the material in material reality, the concept of
"God" is a projection of the personality. The true God, or whatever
we call the ineffable Source, is nonjudgmental, unifying, and loving.
As Yogananda stated, "God is the mirror of silence in which all creation is reflected."

Forgiveness and Response-Ability

It is common in therapeutic circles to hear about the importance
of taking responsibility for your illness or challenging situation.
This attitude has a tendency to create what may be called "new age
guilt" that is disempowering. "I create my own reality and whatever
is happening to me is my fault, so I need to take the blame." How
would taking responsibility for conditions in your life be different
from taking the blame? And what difference does forgiveness make?

Responsibility is how you choose, here and now, to respond to
the circumstances you find yourself in. In the past, circumstances occurred that might have been beyond your control. Consciously
or unconsciously, you chose to interpret those circumstances in a
certain way, which ultimately gave rise to a dysfunctional energy
pattern. Perhaps it was the best choice you could have made, given
the consciousness available to you at that time. There is no blame or
judgment associated with the choice. We're all human; we all have
limitations; we all make mistakes. It is said that, "To err is human,
to forgive is Divine." If we recognize behaviors that no longer serve
us, we can forgive ourselves for making those choices. We can then
choose again.

Responsibility is how you choose, here and now, to respond to the
circumstances you find yourself in.

Then there is the question, where is choice when there is no choice? For example, imagine a young girl who has been sexually abused by her father. Since that incident, she has felt ashamed, guilty and worthless. Her responsibility was not in choosing to be abused. However, once she becomes aware that the way she has held that experience grew out of an unconscious misperception, she can choose again. Her awareness — from an adult perspective — allows her to be "responsible." She is able to respond differently even though she did not as a young child "cause" this to happen to her. While she cannot change what happened then, she can transform her response here and now.

The Holoenergetic Forgiveness Process is particularly effective in restoring her power because the effect of her choice wasn't only psychological. Her experience had a profound and ongoing influence on her, which she holds as an energetic pattern in her body and in the energy field around her. Even if she could go back to the experience and generate compassion for her father, she may not be able to let go of her deep-seated feelings of shame and guilt. She has to access the energetic pattern, resonate with the past experience, bring the moment of choice to conscious awareness, and understand what she really wanted to feel. She can then release the pattern energetically. (This clearing can be done through the Holoenergetic Tracing Process.)

Prior to being conscious of the pattern, she wasn't really responsible for it. However, once she becomes aware of it, she can assume responsibility, in the present, for holding the pattern. Then she can choose to release it. At the same time she may become aware of some resistance to releasing the pattern. She may want to continue to blame, judge and punish the perpetrator, or she may want to remember the abuse so it won't happen again. Once she realizes that holding the trauma of an abusive incident in her body is not the only way to remember and to protect herself, she can choose to release the negative experience energetically. Responsibility always implies choice. Once subconscious choices are identified as such, an individual can take responsibility to choose differently and energetically release the pattern.

That brings us to another question. What if the person who wishes to forgive is still experiencing abuse? If a person is still experiencing abuse, it's not time for forgiveness. It's time for change. It's time to create boundaries or let go of people who are abusive, who drain your life-force energies, or try to control or hurt you. Remember that forgiveness is an internal process and, as such, is self-empowering. Once the external circumstances are changed, you can release any self-judgment, guilt, shame, pain, and conditioned reactivity that you associated with the situation.

If circumstances cannot be changed then, as Christ said, "Forgive them Father, for they know not what they do." Notice that Christ turned to Source when unable to change the external situation. "Not my will, but thy will be done." In this way, he shifted to the greater context of awareness to release personalizing the perpetuation. Perpetrators are unaware that what they do to another, they do themselves. Eventually, they awaken and learn through divine and karmic law to love and forgive themselves and others.

A Doorway to Freedom

Is there a situation or condition in your past that you consider out of your control? Can you recognize that your initial response to the situation was reactive — from pain, hurt, and confusion? You are now free to choose again. This choice point is where the Holoenergetic Forgiveness Process becomes a doorway to freedom, empowerment and true healing.

That is why the most important person to forgive is yourself, including all parts of yourself — the little child, the adolescent/teenager, and the adult. Why all three? Because the "you" you were at each of these ages and stages exists in you as memories, experiences, and energy. As part of the Holoenergetic Forgiveness Process, you will be asked to call forth images of yourself as a child first, then as an adolescent, and finally as an adult. You will be asked to forgive each of the images that represent a portion of your life for which you consciously or subconsciously now feel guilt or shame. You will have an opportunity to communicate things that perhaps you haven't ever consciously accessed before. By releasing any past hurts, you will be inviting all parts of yourself home, reconciling some parts that may have felt separate and alone for a long time. This part of the healing process demonstrates a further level of healing into wholeness.

The most important person to forgive is yourself, including all parts of yourself — the child, the adolescent, and the adult.

There is another aspect to forgiving ourselves at every stage of life. Not only do we forgive ourselves for any perpetrations, real or imagined, we also forgive ourselves for being unloving to ourselves or to others. The key is to feel strongly enough so that you are releasing the stress hormones cortisol and adrenaline. In doing so, we separate the traumatic memory from the emotional charge. While this is a process each individual does for him or herself, imagine the power and release when done individually en masse for some global atrocity, massacre, or holocaust. We collectively might never have to repeat these trauma-inducing patterns again.

Even as we do this process individually, the field is assisting. What Rupert Sheldrake called the morphogenic field — the energetic patterns that many individual habits and actions create in the collective system — is working with us, through us, and for us. You need not feel alone in this process. If you've ever been in a room where a feeling is being accessed collectively — it could be laughter, it could be tears — you know how feelings get amplified, fed back, and reinforced energetically when everyone is in resonance. In the same way, you can walk into a cathedral or holy shrine and sense sacred coherent space.

In the Holoenergetic Forgiveness Process, this entire dialogue occurs silently, inside oneself. This is not "confession;" no external witness is required. No words are spoken aloud. There is no facilitator to judge and no stories to either express or withhold. Because this is an internal dialogue with no one "out there" to explain to or to please, **this is an opportunity to fully feel as much as you possibly can feel.** "Being with" the feelings in the privacy of your own self tends to destabilize the long-term memory. You can then separate out the emotional charge and release it in the presence of a coherent, loving field. The facilitator's job is to create and to hold that transpersonal, nonlocal field.

Everything is made of consciousness and love is consciousness aware of itself.

When suffering is penetrated to its core without attachment, what remains is love. This unconditioned love is a portal to Oneness.

When suffering is penetrated to its core without attachment, what remains is love.

When they hear about the Forgiveness Process, people often say, "Oh, I've done that. I've forgiven my mother, my father, my second grade teacher, my first spouse, etc." What they very likely experienced was the "concept" of forgiveness without any of the emotional fuel needed to truly release the energy held in a past trauma. That's why it is particularly important to focus not just on the person or situation in general, but on specific incidents that trigger emotionally charged memories.

It doesn't matter if you've done forgiveness many times in many different ways. If the issue, whatever it is, still has emotional charge for you, it means you have resisted deep forgiveness until now. What you've been left with is an intellectual concept of forgiveness. So now, in the field of coherence, love, safety and silence... you are ready to free yourself once and for all. Even though you do this process in privacy and silence, you are not alone. Entering into this Holoenergetic Forgiveness Process, you enter a sacred space that holds all the love and coherence of the morphogenic field of Holo-energetic Healing.

THE HOLOENERGETIC FORGIVENESS PROCESS

Before beginning this process, here are some things to remember:

Forgiveness completes your own healing. It releases you from energy patterns that could otherwise contribute to illness and drain your energy.

Remember that forgiving does not mean forgetting. And, it does not mean loving others. That may or may not happen. It just means taking back the energy that you've bound up with feelings you have about certain people and yourself.

Forgiving is "for giving" yourself love and freedom. Please take a moment to decide whom you are now choosing to forgive. It may be one or more individuals other than yourself. (If you are doing the process for the first time, choose just one person other than yourself.)

Note: You might want to record the words that follow in your own voice, and then play the recording back for yourself while you are in a relaxed, meditative state. Be sure to pause at the right times so you allow yourself ample time to experience the process. You can also get a recording of the process at my website www.laskow.net.

- Gently close your eyes and begin to relax, taking slow deep breaths. Allow yourself to relax more and more with each breath. Now just focus on becoming aware of breathing in and breathing out...

- Having decided whom it is you want to forgive, ask yourself honestly if you are really willing to do so now... (pause)
- Take a few more deep slow breaths, relaxing more and more with each exhalation...
- Now, focus attention on your solar plexus in your upper abdomen.
- Draw in a deep breath, as if drawing it through your solar plexus. Hold your breath for a moment, and as you slowly release it, bring to mind by sensing or imagining the image or images of those people you are choosing to forgive. Frame each one in a circle or oval of violet light, like a cameo or portrait.
- Silently communicate to these beings whatever it is they did or did not do that caused you discomfort, stress, or pain. Fully and completely express to each individual anything you have been holding back, be it feelings of hurt, anger, shame, love, sadness, pain, or the desire to blame and punish them. Tell them of specific incidents. Let them know how what they did affected you. Take your time until you feel complete.
- Realize that, in a sense, you have kept the people you have not forgiven imprisoned within you. You have been standing guard just outside the jail door to make sure they do not escape. As their jailer, you have bound yourself to them through your own thoughts and feelings of hurt, blame, and judgment. Forgiveness is a choice to release, to let go of the past, freeing the energy that binds you and blinds you.
- Now, as you look at your willingness to forgive these people...(pause)
- Sense or see yourself standing outside the jail door, about to release them into the light. Forgiveness is an act of self-love. To forgive is not necessarily to forget, or even to love those you've chosen to forgive, but simply to let go of them. This will free up your energy for your own growth, healing, and evolution. Now insert the key of forgiveness into the jail

door, swing it wide open, and prepare to release these beings into the light to go their own way.

- While focusing your attention on the images of those you have chosen to release, take in a deep breath as if through your solar plexus and hold.
- (Read quickly) Completely dissipate these images by forcefully exhaling through your solar plexus NOW. Swirl the energy and release it up into the light.
- Take two more deep breaths, and forcefully exhale through your solar plexus.
- Shift your attention to the center of your chest. Now, gently breathe in and out through your heart center. In the future, whenever you communicate with those you have forgiven, whether verbally or nonverbally, whether they are living or dead, focus your attention on your heart center and speak your truth to them from there.
- If you now choose, silently say what you want to say to these beings from your heart. If you have nothing to say at this time, or when you are finished, you can move on.
- Now bring to your mind, about two feet in front of your heart center, not enclosed in a violet frame, images of yourself, as a child on the left, an adolescent / teenager in the center, and an adult on the right. Silently and with feeling, express to your own images all that you now intend to forgive yourself for. Forgive yourself for all you have done and didn't do as a child, adolescent / teenager, and adult that you now regret. Release all that you have blamed and judged yourself for — all the shame and guilt — all the ways you were unloving to yourself and others. Recall specific incidents. Take your time.
- When you are completely finished, take a deep breath, imagining that you are drawing your breath in through your heart center. As you slowly release your breath from your heart center into the images, feel the forgiveness you have for yourselves.
- Now physically, lovingly embrace the images of yourselves.

Bring them into your heart. Silently tell yourselves:

"I am so sorry you felt separate.

All is forgiven.

And I love you.

Welcome home."

Let yourself feel the love you have for all your selves.

When you are ready, and not before, let your arms come back down. Take as long as you'd like.

Now silently say to yourself:

(Read this slowly, one line at a time, pausing after each line.)

I forgive and release ALL

Past and present, known and unknown

For the highest good of all including myself

I now release all attachment to the past.

I am FREE.

(Always continue with the Unconditional Love Process for Forgiveness.)

UNCONDITIONAL LOVE PROCESS FOR FORGIVENESS

- For a moment become your own best friend and take yourself to the most peaceful place or space you know.

- In the center of your chest, allow yourself to begin to feel a sense of complete and total, boundless, infinite love for yourself — a love for your selves, for your child, adolescent / teenager, and adult. This is a love with no judgments, no comparisons, no attachment to outcome, a love without condition, reason, or cause, beyond all time and space, a love even beyond understanding.

- With your next breath, allow your whole chest to fill with loving light, moving up into your shoulders and down your arms to your fingertips.

- Allow the light to move up into your neck and up into your head, filling your entire head. Imagine this loving light filling your entire head so completely that it begins to flow out the top of your head like a fountain of loving light, cascading down, over and through your body, flowing through your body and out through your feet into the earth below... flowing, clearing, dissolving, and releasing the illusion of separation from your essential nature.

- Now, while focusing your attention on the top of your head, allow yourself to feel the exquisite love that your essential nature has for you — it's expression in form. This is a love that is always present; so you need not learn it or earn it. Just allow yourself to receive it. Sense or imagine a radiant sphere of light six to eight inches above your head. Allow it to slowly descend through the top of your head, down to the center of your chest. Feel yourself radiating with the love your essential nature has for you. Allow its loving light to suffuse your entire body from the top of your head to the tips of your toes, until your body glows with this exquisite love. Allow it in.

- Now ask this exquisite love to:

  Forgive what needs to be forgiven.

  Heal what needs to be healed.

  Do what needs to be done.

  Bring me into wholeness, so that we — the child, adolescent / teenager, and adult — are One.

  (repeat)

  Just ask and then allow it to be done.

  And it is done. You are One — infinitely, eternally, only One.

- Focus again on the center of your chest, feeling that sense of complete, total, boundless infinite love that your essential nature has for you. Now take a deep breath, hold it a moment. When you release your breath, send a burst of light from the center of your chest to every cell, every atom in your body, so that they scintillate and sparkle like stars in the night sky.

- When you are ready, gently open your eyes — at peace — free.

Forgiveness — What It Can and Cannot Do

Having taught this process in many places over the years, I have seen some remarkable healings and transformations take place. Here is a typical story.

One participant from a seminar given in France did the Holoenergetic Forgiveness Process with her mother, with whom she hadn't spoken for quite a while. There had been a lot of acrimony regarding family finances. After we completed the Holoenergetic Forgiveness Process as a group, we had a lunch break. When we returned from the break, the participant shared that she had just received a phone call from her mother who had to track her down by making a number of phone calls. Her mother told her that she'd just decided to settle their disagreements and deposit a significant amount of money in her daughter's bank account. This is one example of the miracle of loving forgiveness.

Another woman — we'll call her Joan — who attended one of my seminars had been estranged from her son. When he got married several years before, he and his new wife inexplicably cut off communication with his entire family. Joan was heartbroken since they had until then been a close-knit family. After some time, she resigned herself to this situation and stopped trying to contact her son. During the seminar, she did the Holoenergetic Forgiveness Process and released her son. Three days later, her son called his sister. They had an hour-long conversation, as if nothing had ever happened.

He has never called any family member again.

Reflecting on the experience, Joan says, "It was a blessing for me to recognize for myself that the Holoenergetic Forgiveness Process absolutely works. I felt utter peace afterward; and, even though he hasn't been in contact since that time, I am free. And so is he."

The Holoenergetic Forgiveness Process is a gateway to transformed relationships... and the primary relationship transformed is with oneself. In freeing herself through the Holoenergetic Forgiveness Process, Joan freed her son as well. For whatever reason, he has chosen to stay separate, and she is at peace with his choice. Her love for him is still in place and is unconditioned. It doesn't require his presence, or for him to be, or not be a certain way.

While it might have been a more satisfying story had the Holo-energetic Forgiveness Process led to a complete reconciliation, perhaps Joan's lesson is a more profound one. Through forgiveness, we free ourselves regardless of what the other person does or doesn't do.

Forgiveness, fully embraced, brings us the gift of freedom, love, and peace.

The freedom, love, and peace that come from forgiveness "passes all understanding." We have no linear, mental, or scientific way to know exactly how it works. Yet experience tells us that forgiveness weaves its magic time after time after time.

One of my practitioners, Ellen, did a forgiveness session with Isabella, an eighty-one-year-old grandmother and great-grand-mother. During the session, Isabella forgave her daughter-in-law and felt a release of tension and a new ease in the relationship. Is-abella then recalled a traumatic incident when she was four or five years old and was on a carousel for the first time. When the carousel stopped and she got off, she was on the opposite side of the carousel and panicked when she didn't see her mother. It was dark, she was lost, and was terrified. From that day forward Isabella had a fear of traveling away from home or on unfamiliar streets and pathways, a fear that remained strong even in later life.

In a letter to Ellen after doing the Holoenergetic Forgiveness Process, she wrote:

> During the Holoenergetic Forgiveness Process, I forgave myself and I realized that there was nothing to be afraid of. I was never alone and I have never been alone. A great power stands to help me at all times, a Divine power; angels help me. I know that I'm never alone, and through this session my heart and my mind were opened and I saw that I never need to be afraid of anything, never need to be afraid of the darkness, never need to be afraid of being lost. Now, after this session I

can go anywhere I want in the city, go to different places, go to different streets, and not be afraid at all! I go now past my limits happily knowing that I will find my way back, and I'm thankful to the power above us, a Supreme Being, for having helped me conquer this fear.

Ellen did a second Holoenergetic Forgiveness Process several weeks later and asked Isabella to share afterward. Isabella said:

I have eleven grandchildren and twenty great-grandchildren. I've always been loved by all of them. They always come close to me. They give me hugs. They give me kisses. They care for me and I feel their love and I love them all, but except this one little child that is my great-grandson. He always seems to look at me and turn away from me as if he doesn't like me…as if I had done something to him…as if I had hurt him. He rejected me. Why? I don't know. I did not force myself on him because I don't believe in that. I love all my descendants, but I wanted them to come freely to me and kiss me and hug me as they so desire. And this little boy, whenever he was around me, he would shy away. He did not want to have anything to do with me. He just looked at me and walked away.

During the Holoenergetic Forgiveness session, Isabella reported:

I talked to him in spirit and I told him to please forgive me if I had done something to him. I loved him and I did not want him to hurt. I don't want to hurt him. I don't want him to feel hurt. I wanted him to come to me and to love me as I love him. And, I care for him very much and I wanted him to feel the love that I have for him. And, I ask for forgiveness and if I had done something to hurt him to please forgive me, and that I forgive whatever had happened between us.

Two days later, Isabella happened to see her great-grandson again. This time, he walked in and without her saying a word, he hugged her, gave her a kiss and said, "Hi, Grandma."

Just like that.

Then he went out to play. Said Isabella:

Later we had lunch and right before he left, again he came over and just gave me a hug without saying a word and I knew everything was well between us. I looked in his eyes and he looked in mine and there was love and forgiveness. It was such a warm feeling that is difficult to express, but in my heart, I know, I know that he has love and he has forgiven me and I know that he loves me as much as I love him. Now there is a beautiful warm feeling for the both of us.

There are many more of these magical forgiveness stories. And yet, none of these stories are as important to you as the forgiveness stories you have yet to experience in your own life. May you use the Holoenergetic Forgiveness Process to heal your world inside and out.

FOR GIVING
LOVE

CHAPTER 6

LIVING IN
WHOLENESS

What you are striving to become is what you already are in essence.
— Ralph Blum

Love is Being aware of One as many.
— Leonard Laskow

Connection becomes attachment through identification with form, with
thoughts, feelings, things and objects. Attachment can be released through
identification with stillness, with Source.
— Leonard Laskow

We have now come full circle.

We began the book focusing on the Game of Awakening, and
now that you have experienced the Holoenergetic Forgiveness Pro-

cess and sampled Holoenergetic Tracing, you are... ahead of the game.

By practicing these heart-focused processes and using the Balancing Breath described later in this chapter, you can integrate wholeness into your life.

When I had the revelation that my work was to heal with love, I initially thought it meant healing at physical, emotional, energetic, and mental levels. Subsequently I realized it was about healing into wholeness, which is ever present. Healing into wholeness is the ultimate medicine. That is why forgiveness brings such peace to those transitioning from form to formlessness. Forgiveness — release of attachment to the past — is completion. In the Vedic tradition — where there is a belief in reincarnation — it is said that the last thing we think of in this life creates the foundation for the next. To be resting in the freedom of forgiveness, surrounded by love, allows easier release of the body into the realm of formless consciousness. That is why forgiveness is such a valuable tool for practitioners working with those who are dying.

Healing into wholeness is the ultimate medicine.

When forgiveness dissolves separation from your inner light, what remains is love. When loving awareness flows through the heart, it shifts and coheres the vibration of the inner energy body into resonance with your essential nature. You align with the truth of who you really are and the truth of what is. That is why the Conscious Heart Focus presented in chapter 2 is a sustaining practice for living in wholeness.

Conscious Heart Focus

Try these three simple steps of the Conscious Heart Focus now, even while reading.

1. **Shift** your attention from wherever it is now to the center of your chest.
2. **Breathe** in and out as if through the center of your chest for at least three breaths.
3. **Focus** on something that always opens your heart, makes you feel good, and brings a smile to your heart. Switch your attention to the feel-good channel.

Not only does this simple process bring peace to your body and mind, it is also a gateway to stillness beyond this world. Beyond the physical, in the unmanifest, we live a parallel existence in which we are all interconnected. At the physical level we are only aware of the five senses and three dimensions (four, if we include time). When we experience only three dimensions with our physical senses, we appear separate, isolated, alone. When we see through the lens of the heart, as we do through the Conscious Heart Focus, we see and feel the interconnectedness. We feel love; we feel unity; we feel wholeness.

Along with the Conscious Heart Focus, living in wholeness implies the practice of presence.

From Duality to Unity
— the Practice of Presence

The heart resolves duality into unity.

Since the brain and mind attempt to organize chaos by excluding unmanifest space and formlessness, and the heart resolves duality into unity, how do we divest from the divisive conversations of the mind and invest in the unity of the heart? How do we transcend the exclusions of our neurobiology and bring forth the inclusiveness of the heart that recognizes formless interconnectedness?

We do so by practicing presence and accessing what we call the Aware Witness. Although this book is about forgiveness, unconditioned love, and freedom, once the Holoenergetic Forgiveness Process has taken place, we can perpetuate that love and freedom through the Aware Witness.

To prepare to function from the Aware Witness, let's review perception from the perspective of the Bucket Process from chapter 3. While we'd like to imagine our perceptions are clean, clear, and accurate representations of "what is," there is the matter of our prior conditioning, experiences, and beliefs that serve as an invisible filter. To paraphrase Albert Einstein, a problem cannot be solved at the same level of consciousness in which it was created. To accurately interpret our perceptions requires a step upward to a higher, more expansive consciousness. At this level of integrated consciousness, in the Bucket Process, we recognize that both hands are relatively "right" about their perceptions of water temperature. Taken from a more expanded awareness, we have a more complete view of what's so.

The transformational process of healing requires a shift to a higher dimension of consciousness. At this higher level, we can experience even pain as bigger than the disruptive physical signal that has gotten our attention. When we become aware of the "space" in which the pain occurs, we can extract the full meaning of the painful experience. Instead of resisting the pain, we unconditionally accept its presence. This acceptance becomes the space or context in which we hold the pain. Pain is the content arising in that space of expanded presence. By focusing attention on the space (the context) — the expanded awareness in which the pain arises — the pain diminishes.

You may be familiar with the remarkable story of Jack Schwarz, who was being held and tortured at a Nazi prison camp during World War II. At one point, he was tortured until he became unconscious. While unconscious, he spontaneously experienced an expanded awareness of Oneness in which he realized that the man torturing him was torturing himself. Upon regaining consciousness, he said to his torturer, from this expanded Oneness, "I love you." At that instant his wounds began to heal miraculously. The prison guards never tortured him again. In later life, he demonstrated what seemed to be a super-human ability to transcend pain and to heal. For example, he could stick a large needle through his arm, feel no pain, and have no bleeding.

Here's something you can try yourself, right now. Press the area between your thumb and forefinger until it feels painful. You won't have to press too hard. Now, instead of focusing on the pain, expand your focus to the space surrounding the pain. You will find that the pain diminishes, even if you press harder. This is another example of the power of focusing on context (space) rather than content (the physical area where pain is occurring).

And what would happen if, instead of focusing on context, you were to focus "totally" on the content, the form arising in the present, without denying, resisting or repressing it? What would happen if you were to focus on the source of the form?

Diving into the essence of the form by unconditionally accepting what is so is ultimately the same as transcending the form. Dive into fear, anger, shame, pain or sadness and follow it back to its source. It is all consciousness temporarily assuming this feeling form — a wave in the ocean of consciousness.

(For example, Surfers don't try to paddle away from big waves. They dive into the wave or they surf it.)

So, instead of repressing, denying or resisting what is, dive directly into the form that arises. All form is perceived and experienced through the mind, and the mind is a creation of consciousness. So when you dive into the consciousness-created mind to discover the source of suffering, the suffering dissolves into consciousness itself.

Everything is made of consciousness, and love is consciousness aware of itself.

When suffering is penetrated to its core without attachment, what remains is love. This unconditioned love is a portal to Oneness.

Look carefully at the picture below. If you look at it one way, appears to be a young maiden, and if you look at it another way, it becomes an old woman's profile. When people look at it, they can only see one of these images at a time, even when they know the ambiguous drawing shows two distinct images. Psychologists and experts on visual perception confirm this — you can see only one image or another at one time, not both.

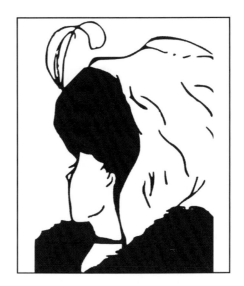

This is an example of the limitations of sense perceptions in providing comprehensive information. Looking at the drawing, our sense perception sees either the maiden or the crone but doesn't see both simultaneously. This either / or way of seeing may be the nervous system's way of avoiding overload and organizing chaos. However, even though we can only see one or the other in a given moment, we are "aware" that both exist simultaneously. This simultaneous awareness, when focused on both the form and the formless, is the basis of the spiritual dictum that essence is form, and form is essence.

So — back to the buckets in chapter 3 — when you put your hand in the hot water and then in the tepid, it is cool; and if you put your hand in the ice water and then put it in the center bucket, it is warm. Each of these feels "absolute" — you cannot experience both states at the same time at the level of perception. Given the limitations and omissions of the senses, the Aware Witness becomes a far more accurate "witness" in any situation.

The Aware Witness

In my seminars we begin most exercises with the Grounding, Aligning, and Centering Process (presented at the end of chapter 3). We ground to the earth, align with soul and Spirit, and center ourselves in the heart space that resolves all seeming duality into unity. This is the way we begin to practice presence.

As we said earlier, the mind and its extensions — the senses — do not unite. They are both designed to ensure survival and organize chaos by excluding seeming contradiction and space. The mind and senses put perceptions and experiences in compartments for purposes of pattern recognition. So unity is not accessed through the mind. Time appears to be another way of organizing chaos. It allows us to sequence our activities rather than having the chaotic overwhelm of having everything happen at once. To get the truly higher, broader, and deeper perspective requires timelessness by practicing presence through the Aware Witness portal.

The mind and senses are both designed to ensure survival and organize chaos by excluding seeming contradiction and space.

We cultivate the Aware Witness by stilling the mind so that a higher voice can be heard, and we can access a more expansive con-

text. Psalm 46:10 tells us, "Be still and know that I am God." In
stillness, by quieting the mind, we unite with what we call God and
experience Presence. This same stillness also allows us access to
what Ramana Maharshi called "the silence of the cave of the heart"
— the embodiment of unitive love. Being still is being one with God
or Spirit.

Just for a minute, tune into the thoughts going through your
head. Chances are they are about categorization and duality, constantly contrasting "mine" and "not mine," and "sorting" reality on
the basis of either survival / loss or personal benefit / gain. This is
good for me, that is not good for me.

Sorting by the ego's criteria is a helpful way of functioning when
we seek "translational" change or healing that shifts energy and attention from one thing to another on the material plane. However, the truth beyond duality can only be "heard" through quieting
the chatter of the mind. By accessing this transpersonal witness,
we are liberated from the trance of personality and tuned into the
ever-present nonlocal field.

The Holoenergetic Forgiveness Process, at its best, helps us to
transform a painful situation or memory we've been holding on to
by taking us to a transcendent space. Practicing presence through
the processes and exercises described and reviewed in this chapter
can make this boundless field of Oneness more familiar and more
easily accessible. In the space of Aware Witness, we become aware
of both the experience and "noticer" of the experience we wish to
forgive and release.

Being in these two places at once is what allows us to fully experience all the feelings bundled in the original traumatic event. At the
same time, we can be in the transcendent space where those feelings
are seen as temporal events arising in the larger awareness. Holding
and feeling the feelings of separation while in a place of unity desta-
bilizes and discharges the emotionally charged long-term memory.
The long-term memory then reconfigures in the hippocampus so
that the recollections are now free of emotional reactivity. As we
experience this sense of One Consciousness, we return to the place

we started in the unmanifest and recognize that we have been "here" all along.

Keep in mind there is nothing "wrong" or "bad" or unnatural about feeling the feelings of separation. The material world naturally takes us into differentiation, which we misinterpret as separation. That is the experience of life in the third dimension. When we hold the simultaneous awareness of the greater truth of our Being, the Aware Witness reminds us that Oneness is ever present, beyond the boundaries of space, time and matter. When we realize that even apparent separation is contained in Oneness, we can rise above the "game board" only to return again from this expansive consciousness to play a happier, more joyful game, seeing it without attachment for the game it is.

Content, Context and the Noticer

You've probably noticed that the "content" of life has gotten vastly more complex over the course of your lifetime. At a time when content can be overwhelming, "context" becomes even more important. The dictionary defines context as "the circumstances that form the setting for an event, statement, or idea, and in terms of which it can be fully understood and assessed." Again — paraphrasing Einstein — on the level of circumstances, the condition cannot be transformed. Only by shifting to a "context" that offers a more comprehensive point of view can the content be integrated and released.

The real "secret" is this: Unconditioned love is not about changing the content of your life. It's about accessing the ever-present context in which all content arises and subsides. When we find this context within, the search for love from the outside ends. Non-conditioned love is the ocean of awareness we tap into when we practice presence.

Suffering is experienced when we identify with the content of love — the people, places, objects, conditions that we associate with our happiness. We free ourselves from suffering when we remember that non-conditioned love is the context of "all things." When we experience content through this context, we experience peace, freedom, and unity.

Non-conditioned love is the context of all things.

To reiterate what we said before, there is a difference between "unconditioned love" and "non-conditioned love." You can focus unconditioned love like a vector toward a person, place, or object without condition or expectation. Non-conditioned love simply IS and has no specific object. Rather than focusing, it radiates like the sun. This state of non-conditioned love is context, is Being, without identification or attachment.

In ordinary life, we experience all content through a context. Usually, this context is the smaller "personality me." The ordinary contextual question we ask is, "Is this good / bad for me?" While this discernment is convenient for navigating the choices of everyday life, when we live from this ordinary and limiting context, we subject ourselves to suffering whenever reality doesn't meet our conditions.

Whenever we make our love about some "thing" (i.e., something manifest on the material plane), we forget that, in essence, we are that non-conditioned love. There is nothing wrong with "horizontal" love within duality, directed toward other people, places and things. However, the boundless peace that comes from "vertical" love, like the sun, shines equally on all. Non-conditioned love transcends suffering because it doesn't identify with anything or anyone as the source of our happiness. Vertical love is the love that extends from duality to Unity, that aligns Spirit with matter, essence with form — spontaneously taking us beyond the relatedness of duality into wholeness.

Most of the time when we talk about love, we are talking about relatedness. We want to connect with, merge with another individual, beloved place, or activity. This is horizontal love because it involves some "other" within duality. Non-conditioned "vertical" love spontaneously resolves all duality into Unity. There is no other, only One.

From this context of ever-present non-conditioned love, we can appreciate the paradoxical nature of existence — ever changing, same as always. Consciousness turned outward through attention and intention creates the world of form — i.e., content. Consciousness turned inward dissolves all content into the formless One.

Included in "content" is the content of our minds. When we transcend content, we experience the peace that passes all understanding — and the love without an object, cause, or reason. In this space of profound epiphany, we experience no needing and no wanting. We already ARE everything, and love is the context that holds all content.

Again, all suffering is content. Hurt, pain, longing … these are all about objects, the content in our lives. The same is true for pleasure. Pleasure can be conditional and fleeting, dependent upon conditions "out there." Beyond pain or pleasure, beyond joy or sadness, the context of non-conditioned love opens to boundless freedom and peace.

When you practice forgiveness through the Holoenergetic Forgiveness Process, you access this greater context to process the content that is the object of your distress. Forgiveness is a tool of the soul that allows you to manifest simultaneous awareness, and instead of merely noticing your distress, you notice who is doing the noticing, returning you to wholeness.

To sustain the ever-present context of Oneness in our ordinary reality, I have developed some processes that we use in our seminars. I will outline some of these exercises here and later in the chapter.

ACCESSING HEAD HEART SPACE

To gain entry to ever-present context, a foundational first step is to learn how to access the head / heart space.

Read over the steps first so that you understand what to do.

Head Space

1. Gently close your eyes and become aware of your breath breathing itself.
2. When you open your eyes, focus your attention on an object in the room, not a person.
3. As you look at the object, see it as if you are seeing it for the first time without thinking about it, naming or labeling it. Just look.
4. Now, while looking at it pull your attention and your breath inward toward the space inside the back of your head. Just have the intention and your consciousness will find its way into your head space.
5. As best you can, notice the space.
6. Now, from this space, notice the object.
7. The object is in the foreground, and the space is the background.
8. What do you notice?

Heart Space

1. Gently close your eyes and become aware of your breath breathing itself.
2. Sense or imagine breathing in and out as if through the center of your chest, your energetic heart, for at least three breaths.
3. When you open your eyes, focus your attention on the same object without thinking about it or naming it. Just look.
4. Now, while looking at it, pull your attention and breath inward into the space inside the back of your heart. Just have the intention and your consciousness will find its way into your heart space.
5. As best you can, notice the space.
6. Now, from this space, notice the object.
7. When you allow yourself to unconditionally, nonjudgmentally accept the object exactly as it is, what do you notice?

This space in the head and the heart is the unconditioned space prior to thinking that we all share — a space of unity, a space of truth, a space of love. This is the background space that never changes — that aspect of the Aware Witness that remains constant regardless of the ever-changing foreground perceptions of objects and forms.

The difference that people frequently report between the head and heart space has to do with the distortions of accessibility. Access to the head space is most readily distorted by conditioned thinking while access to the heart space is most readily distorted by conditioned feelings and emotions.

Using the Holoenergetic Forgiveness Process and Unconditional Love Process for Forgiveness potentially provides you with the tools for accessing the undistorted head space and heart space. Then, the truth of "what is" is directly seen, and the space of unity with "what is" is directly felt.

Most people who do this process report a felt sense of oneness or connectedness with the object that they didn't have the first time they looked at it. Others have an expanded sense of other people in the room. Some even experience the space between themselves and the object beginning to vibrate, which is a perception of coherent loving energy. This space of expanded awareness can be called the "noticer," the Aware Witness, or the soul. In this space, we become simultaneously aware of the object and the "noticer." If we were to then turn our attention inward, even the noticer dissolves into the ocean of awareness. There is no longer a subject or an object, just pure existence.

Let's explore this noticer, this observer self — what we call in this book the Aware Witness — a bit more carefully. The Aware Witness is the editor of our projections and knows we can change the filters we have used to interpret our sensory information and "make the movies" we project and live. The Aware Witness knows present perceptions we now hold energetically as geometric patterns in our minds can be transformed by altering previous information and experiences. While our beliefs and attitudes "select" which perceptions come into our foreground, it's the Aware Witness — our observer self — that perceives "what is" most directly.

The Aware Witness allows us to see the thoughts, feelings, seeming paradoxes, separation, and illness or disease from a perspective that can then be incorporated, integrated, and resolved. Healing occurs as we dissolve our illusions of separateness and move toward wholeness. In this movement toward wholeness, our Aware Witness is not only a helper but also a model, allowing us to sense our full potential, the whole that is greater than the sum of the parts. The shift to the context of the Aware Witness is a major step toward wholeness, which is the essence of our healing work.

Healing occurs as we dissolve our illusions of separateness and move toward wholeness.

The Aware Witness is also the gateway to our sixth sense, intuition. The deeper we go into the healing process, the more it serves to draw upon our intuitive sense and the more useful it becomes to shift our consciousness at will. It's best to be able to simultaneously identify with the part of us that experiences the contractive circumstance, and at the same time step outside of that circumstance to make new, more expansive choices. These choices integrate content and context, as can happen in the Holoenergetic Tracing and Forgiveness Processes. Paradoxically, we first need to identify with our thoughts, feelings, and sensations to then be able to dis-identify with them by shifting our focus to the larger context that contains them. In other words, it's important to accept or resonate with what is on the one hand, and to simultaneously understand it as what appears to be. Think back to the bucket experiment. The "hands" understood the water temperature as either hot or cold. This simultaneous awareness of both hot and cold depends on shifting to the contextual awareness that recognizes prior conditioning.

Thus, the healing process involves both identification and dis-identification. Identification allows hurts and attachments to completely come to the surface so they can be accepted, felt, and released. Repressing these by "trying to think positive" actually thwarts genuine healing and release because it prevents the aware feeling of separation that is required to experience that separation in the ultimate context of connectedness.

When your feelings of separation are fully present in your awareness, you can understand and accept them. Then you can take the next step — releasing identification and shifting to the Aware Witness. This shift can be likened to taking in the view from the top of a mountain after a long climb. The air is fresh and clear. From this "higher ground," you can look around and observe your patterns as if you were looking down at the camp from which you've just come.

Here is another paradox of "identification." While identifying with one's own personality is a cause of suffering, identifying with another through the heart is the gateway to compassion. Buddha taught that in order to understand the object of our perception we have to be one with it (e.g., "walking in another's shoes"). This "felt awareness" can be called loving identification. Through loving identification, I become you, so I understand you. I see and feel what you see and feel, and I understand. I understand why you are as you are and what you really want. Ultimately, your behavior was either a call for love or an expression of love.

Interestingly, we can also identify with another through the solar plexus. We call this "sympathy" — which can activate our own past memories and distress. Sympathy in this way can distort our perceptions, allow us to be manipulated or manipulate, and leave us burdened with another person's pain. When we identify through the heart — "compassion" — our personal agenda disappears, separation dissolves, and we have unconditioned compassion. When the force of compassion and understanding becomes a living, healing force in our lives, it becomes wisdom. Wisdom is the compassionate realization of truth.

Wisdom is the compassionate realization of truth.

When we understand another through the cognitive mind, we call this "empathy." In other words, we experience compassion from the heart, empathy from the head, and sympathy from the solar plexus.

Transforming something in your life requires you to dis-identify, to step outside of it and become "observer-participant." You become an aware loving witness who participates and interacts. You release yourself from personal identification while you hold the expanded understanding you gained through the identification.

Dis-identification is like a fulcrum — the still point of the Aware Witness that allows your will to act as a lever, to shift or change that with which you identify. Put another way, it's hard to move a rock when you're standing on it. But, if you step aside and use a lever with the fulcrum, you can move even heavy stones. The lever is your will, intention, and imagery… AND it needs the fulcrum of dis-identified aware understanding (via the still point of the Aware Witness) to be most effective.

So, why not just step off the rock and let it be?

Because merely stepping off the rock is to disconnect, to detach, to separate from, or to deny its existence. When you dis-identify rather than deny, you step off with a higher understanding of the context and the intent to change. In Unfolding Self, Molly Brown comments: "As we become more aware, as we learn to observe without judgment… we move into the more subtle state of Being: aware of awareness, becoming aware of that which is aware, the self." When we change our point of view this way, we can get to the core issues or original source of the pain; we can know what is beyond the distortions of our senses, feelings and beliefs. As the Aware Witness we dis-identify from our perceptual limitations.

Ideally, in the Resonance, Release, and Reformation phases of healing, the Aware Witness is primarily transpersonal, able to shift awareness and perceive a truth beyond the perspectives of the physical, emotional, and mental self. As with the bucket experiment, the Aware Witness not only knows what the hands are experiencing, but it also knows the origin or context of that experience. When we have a disease or illness, it is easy to focus on the single reality of the disease to define us. It's similar to how each hand defines the water temperature; each hand separately "knows" it is right about the temperature, and therefore the other hand must be wrong. This is an either / or way of interpreting experience, which crystalizes beliefs that sustain wounds and suffering.

Frequently when we are ill, there's a part of us that feels contracted or separate and "knows" it is "right" about its experience. When we experience through this contracted filter, all of the "facts" seem to support our position. But, to paraphrase Frank Lloyd Wright, truth is more important than fact. Only at the level of the Aware Witness, when we take into account the origin and meaning of the illness and the beliefs that created the illusion of separation, can the paradox of illness be resolved. I say "paradox" because behind all illness lies a positive life force that has become thwarted and distorted in its expression.

The Ever-present Context of the Soul

I define soul as "the awareness that simultaneously recognizes our individuality and our unity and merges the two as its purpose." Soul is the simultaneous awareness of form and essence. Soul is the conscious witness of both uniqueness and unity and is felt as the energy of love. As my friend Asandra has expressed it, "The soul imbued with desire seeks its own awakening."

If we imagine pure existence as white light, and physicality as a prism, when we take physical form our "unique soul print" is expressed as a series of color frequencies on a rainbow spectrum. Put another way, we are simultaneously unique and part of the whole. As separate differentiated individuals, we express a group of "frequencies" that are our unique vibration. As such we are a divine fractal of all that is.

We are simultaneously unique and universal.

So why is this important?

What we call the soul is our gateway, our connection, our reminder of Universal Unconditioned Love. We experience the soul in daily life when, through the Aware Witness, we access this felt sense of uniqueness and unity. Being in the Aware Witness, we allow the light of this love to shine on whatever human situation we seek to heal, transform, or transcend.

The soul then is the mediator between subject and object, the context that is ever-present, regardless of the content. The Holoenergetic Forgiveness Process calls forth the soul as the coherent space of freedom and unconditioned self-acceptance. As we learn to use the Holoenergetic Forgiveness Process whenever we become aware of a shadow blocking the light in life, we begin living in and from our soul more frequently. From this higher perspective, we find ourselves less prone to upset. And, without the distortions of distress, the calling of our soul is more clearly heard.

A friend recently shared with me her concern that her mother was having short–term memory loss, but she also noticed that there was a benefit to these lapses of memory. "These days," she said, "when my mother gets angry and begins to fume at something she has taken offense to, I just wait a few minutes and she forgets what is making her angry. Then all that is left is the energy of anger, which quickly dissipates without the memory of the cause."

The Standing Wave
— How Thoughts Create Reality

In the study of energy systems, when a wave of a particular frequency and amplitude meets a wave of the same frequency and amplitude coming from the opposite direction, a standing wave occurs at the point where they meet and resonate. The patterns created by the two waves at this juncture then become self-organizing; that is, this standing wave becomes a template that tends to seek like forms and perpetuate itself.

Using the pipe organ as an example, the length and size of the pipe determines the form of the standing wave. When air is pumped through the pipe, it sets up a standing wave characteristic of that form, which we experience as sound. When frequencies merge to create resonant standing waves, geometric energy patterns or templates are formed. These templates are capable of storing and transmitting information to other forms that resonate with them. Hence, the other familiar example of tuning forks tuned to the same frequency vibrating together when one is hit.

Furthermore, when the left and right hemispheres of the brain come into synchrony, they energetically fuse to create a standing wave form that resonates with the transpersonal space. The resulting unity shifts our perceptions from the body-mind realm to the spiritual realm. In other words, when these two hemispheres are in harmony, through our own attunement, we have access to the higher vibrations of soul and Spirit. In contrast, when we are in distress, that too sets up a vibration, and the distressed vibration is likewise a magnetic attractor for people, situations, and things that resonate with that "less than" state.

Within the energetic model of Holoenergetic Healing, beliefs, thoughts, and feelings have energetic signatures. For example, a particular individual's feeling of not being good enough would have a specific, recognizable form that is as unique to that person as his or her handwritten signature. When we believe or feel something, that belief or feeling creates a specific energetic form. That form exists within the energy field of our own body-mind and can also extend outward. This vibration becomes our radar system seeking and / or creating matching forms to resonate with in the external world. So, if you've wondered why you or someone else continue to create and recreate the same kinds of conditions and relationships in life (same plot, different cast of characters), it is likely due to the signal being broadcast.

The energetic templates or holoforms of our thoughts and feelings seek out circumstances (other people, experiences, physical forms, etc.) that are supportive of these templates. That is, the energetic forms of our own beliefs, thoughts, and feelings tend to find other people or situations that confirm, validate, prove, or justify them. If our energy configures as a victim "form," we'll tend to gravitate toward circumstances that make it appear that the world is our victimizer. If our energy takes a more active and self-actualizing form, we will tend to magnetize circumstances filled with opportunity and resources. The resonance between the external world and the forms established within our own energy fields creates what we perceive as our individual reality.

The resonance between the external world and the forms established within our own energy fields creates what we perceive as "reality."

In Holoenergetic Healing, we use breathing to focus and amplify attention so as to align with our transpersonal nature. Conscious breathing reinforces the new forms we choose by creating a standing wave resonance (organizing energy field) within us that attracts to itself, from the world around us, forms like itself.

For example, we might have a fear of intimacy that we want to heal because we have met someone with whom we would like to share a long-term relationship. We begin with the desire to change the energy pattern that expresses that fear. Then, we discover the traumatic origin and the positive life-force energy behind the fear. We create the mental image of the new form where we see ourselves as freely receiving and giving love. However, just having created that new form is not enough. We must then align with the life-force energies of our soul, commit our will to maintain the new form, and focus our intention to establish a plan to express this new form. The new template becomes a magnetic energy field that attracts like forms from the world around us. The Holoenergetic Tracing Process is designed to facilitate this radical transformation. The Intuitive Co-Creator Process (in the appendix) helps manifest what is wanted once you release the old forms.

At each step — from formulating the desire to making a mental image, accessing soul, developing a plan, etc. — we use the breath to focus and to amplify our endeavor. Conscious breathing animates and amplifies the new form. Conscious breath sparks the energy to change both the inner and outer states toward our desired reality.

Conscious breathing also helps us to balance the hemispheres of our brain. We create a sense of unity within as we inhale the "inspirational" breath of life and exhale the "expiration" of the old. Taking in the new life energies and letting go of that which is ready to die, we balance other polarities — the active and passive, the sympathetic and the parasympathetic, the masculine and feminine — through our rhythmic patterns of breathing. We balance the hemispheres of our brain with the Balancing Breath (see below). This state of consciousness coheres both hemispheres and profoundly facilitates the healing process.

The Balancing Breath
— Portal to the Aware Witness

While doing research at a Northern California University biofeedback laboratory on the relationship of breath to brain wave activity, I discovered a breathing technique that I found to be of great value in healing work. I call this as the Balancing Breath because it allows us to rapidly expand and elevate consciousness by synchronizing the right and left hemispheres of the brain, bringing the mind into a state of resonant coherence.

As part of my early research, I explored an ancient Yogic technique for balancing the brain hemispheres. This technique, called "alternate-nostril breathing," involves alternately pinching and releasing the nostrils with the fingers while breathing, first inhaling on one side, then exhaling on the other.

I did this exercise while being monitored by an electro-encephalograph (EEG), which measured activity in the right and left hemispheres of my brain. I noticed that using my hand to perform the alternate-nostril breathing technique as described by the yogis, created an unbalanced hemispheric pattern. (Neurologically, the contralateral hemisphere of the brain was stimulated.) However, when I kept my hands relaxed in my lap and simply imagined air moving in one nostril, then out the other, and so on, something interesting occurred. The EEG showed that the right and left hemispheres of my brain came into synchrony producing what is referred to as hemispheric coherence. My brainwave activity displayed a synchronous Alpha brain wave pattern (about 7-8 cps) for both hemispheres.

This state of resonance, brought about through the balancing breath, enhances performance on many levels. Balanced breath is especially valuable for healing work. Since it may be challenging — at least initially — to stay in the state of balanced hemispheric coherence for long periods of time, the Balancing Breath is most effective when practiced just before healing yourself and others, as preparation for meditation or for accessing the Aware Witness.

There are several ways breathing brings us into balance. Rhythmic, even breathing can balance the autonomic nervous system because inhalation arouses sympathetic nervous system activity while exhaling elicits parasympathetic activity. Breathing in through one nostril and out through the other adds another level of balance. This hemispheric balance is known in the East as the balance of yin and yang.

How does your body accomplish such a balance?

In your natural automatic breathing pattern, the airflow through one nostril predominates for about ninety minutes. At that point, a switch occurs and the airflow is greater through the other nostril for the next ninety minutes. You can determine which nostril you're primarily breathing through by wetting the palm of your hand and breathing into it to determine which side is cooler. Or, you can compress each nostril while breathing in to determine which is easier to breathe through.

The switch in nostril dominance every ninety minutes is mediated by the hypothalamus, which essentially controls the autonomic nervous system. The sympathetic portion of the autonomic nervous system causes the blood vessels that supply the mucous membranes in the nasal passages to constrict; the parasympathetic portion causes them to dilate. This rhythmic constriction and dilation is experienced as dominance of one passage or another.

Nasal dominance can have a significant effect on our thinking as well as on our moods and our state of consciousness. When we breathe in through the left nostril, the right-brain hemisphere is stimulated. Conversely, when we breathe in through the right nostril, the left-brain hemisphere is stimulated. D. A. Werntz, a researcher at the University of California at San Diego School of Medicine, demonstrated that breathing through one nostril generated EEG activity in the opposite brain hemisphere.

Nasal dominance can have a significant effect on our thinking as well as on our moods and our state of consciousness.

This is important because the right and left hemispheres of the brain have different functions. Characteristically the left hemisphere is associated with verbal, linear, rational activities while the right hemisphere is generally associated with spatial, nonlinear, intuitive activities. Werntz's research showed that when we consciously use one nostril or another dominantly, the task performance associated with that side is enhanced. Right nostril breathing, for instance, improved the verbal skills associated with the left hemisphere, while left nostril breathing improved the intuitive or spatial skills associated with the right hemisphere.

You can change dominance, regardless of which side is dominant at the moment, by directing or imagining breath coming in through the opposite nostril. If, for instance, you want to stimulate more intuitive activity, you can start breathing in through your left nostril several times by compressing the right nostril, or by simply imagining your breath coming in through your left nostril.

David S. Shannahoff-Khalsa, a colleague of Werntz's, found that appetite and digestion are enhanced during right nostril/left brain dominance. He also points out that left nostril emphasis is more beneficial for receiving new ideas, while right nostril emphasis facilitates speaking abilities. Nostril dominance likewise impacts our autonomic nervous system so that not only one side of the brain, but one side of the entire body, will have greater sympathetic activity at any given time.

Studies with volunteers have shown that when blood is drawn from each arm at regular intervals, the level of norepinephrine produced by the sympathetic nervous system is always significantly higher on the side correlating with nostril dominance. This demonstrates that the body, as well as the brain switches dominance at regular intervals.

By breathing through both nostrils simultaneously after the Balancing Breath, you can further balance the two hemispheres of the brain and the functions associated with them. Breathing through both nostrils at the same time may also help generate natural crossover of dominance. When a ninety-minute cycle ends, it takes about ten minutes for a nostril dominance to change naturally from one side to the other. This crossover correlates with peak task performance of the skills associated with both hemispheres and the balanced nostril dominance. By breathing through both nostrils simultaneously, you can induce this optimal crossover state at will.

Normally, we achieve a balance between the two hemispheres over a period of time. The Balancing Breath practice can help you achieve this balance intentionally. This is particularly helpful before and during meditation, healing, or counseling to shift consciousness into the transpersonal dimension.

THE BALANCING BREATH PROCESS

As you do this exercise, try to involve as many senses as you can. For example, as you breathe in, focus on your nostril and notice that the air flowing through your nostril feels cool. Notice how it feels warmer in your nostrils as you exhale. As you breathe, air moves the tiny hairs that line your nasal passages. Allow yourself to sense these movements.

You might also imagine that you are breathing in light or color, or even a fragrance, such as that of a rose. Or you can breathe in the seven chakra colors: red, orange, yellow, green, blue, indigo and violet, ensuring the seven cycles, which help to balance your entire subtle energy system. I call this "the rainbow breath."

What is exciting about the Balancing Breath is that it enables you to make one brain hemisphere more dominant or bring both hemispheres and your autonomic nervous system into balance as you choose. Through your breathing, you can consciously influence your body, your feelings, and your thoughts to shift your state of consciousness. The Balancing Breath links the physical body with spirit, and, in so doing, it helps to bring healing into the realm of conscious choice.

- Assume a comfortable, relaxed position and gently close your eyes.
- Exhale, allowing your lungs to empty and relax.
- As you breathe in, imagine your breath coming in through your left nostril and hold it for a moment.
- As you exhale, imagine your breath coming out your right

nostril. Breathe as described for seven cycles, alternating the nostrils on the in breath. (Each inhalation followed by an exhalation is one complete cycle.)

- On your eighth cycle, breathe in through both nostrils simultaneously up into the center of your head. Hold that breath for a moment and focus your attention on the center of your forehead.
- Release your breath as if you were exhaling it through your forehead. This opens up the energy center associated with the intuitive functions of your mind.
- On your ninth cycle, breathe in through both nostrils simultaneously. Hold that breath for a moment and focus your attention on the space inside the back of your head.
- Release your breath as if you were exhaling it into the space inside the back of your head. This opens up the third ventricle of your brain, the primary conduit for higher guidance beyond mind.
- On your tenth cycle, breathe in through both nostrils simultaneously. Hold that breath for a moment and focus your attention on the top of your head. Release your breath as if you were exhaling through the top of your head. This opens the energy center associated with unitive awareness and non- local interconnectedness.
- Remain open, present and aware as you continue to breathe through both nostrils simultaneously. (Note: The Aware Witness is a space, not a location, and as such can be accessed through many portals. When using the Balancing Breath, the Aware Witness can be accessed through intuitive knowing or higher guidance, as well as unitive awareness.)

When both hemispheres are brought into balance, as happens with the Balancing Breath, consciousness is shifted into the transpersonal dimension. This balanced and synchronous state may be accompanied by a release of energy, sometimes seen as light. The release of energy may be sensed as a blue light. In the Eastern traditions, the light is sometimes referred to as the Blue Pearl.

When both hemispheres are brought into balance, consciousness shifts into the transpersonal dimension.

As I explored the Balancing Breath, I realized that when I saw the Blue Pearl, there had been a subtle energetic fusion of my right and left hemispheres. Along with the light, I experienced a sense of inner peace and unity. My consciousness at that moment seemed to expand to include an area just above my head, which is often referred to as the "transpersonal space," "soul space," or crown chakra.

In this inclusive state of consciousness, it became obvious to me that it takes energy to maintain the illusion of separation, just as it takes energy to maintain the separation of charge across the cell membrane or in a battery. Therefore, when whatever is held to be separate is unified, energy is released. This is the energy of synergy, the energy of the unified whole that is greater than the sum of its parts. To the extent that we open ourselves to the transpersonal realms of consciousness — through such activities as meditation and conscious breathing or using the Conscious Heart Focus Process — the energy we use to maintain the illusion of separation is no longer needed, and the separation energy is released as light.

In ordinary states of consciousness, where one brain hemisphere or the other is dominant, it is easier to maintain the illusion of separation. This illusion may cause us to feel alienated from our center or Source. We can experience this separation as a fear of loss or abandonment. We feel out of touch with our true nature. We are not in resonance with our own bodies, our own minds, or our own selves. Nor are we in a resonant relationship with the universe.

Conversely, in those moments when we experience oneness and come into alignment with our true nature, we no longer feel alone or abandoned. We are coming home, in resonance with Source. If we remain misaligned or separated from Source, we eventually become ill, which reminds us to come back into resonant unity. The essence of healing, then, is to become one with the Source of our being.

I like the way the Gospel of Thomas addresses the illusion of separation and duality in relation to the unity of matter and spirit:

> *Jesus saw children who are being suckled.*
> *He said to his disciples:*
> *These children who are being suckled*
> *are like those who enter the Kingdom.*
>
> *They said unto him:*
> *Shall we then, being children,*
> *enter the kingdom?*
>
> *Jesus said to them:*
> *When you make the two one,*
> *and when you make the inner as the outer*
> *And the outer as the inner,*
> *And the above as the below,*
>
> *And when you make*
> *the male and the female into a single one,*
> *So that the male will not be male*
> *and a female not be female,*
> *Then shall you enter the Kingdom.*
>
> *(Gospel of Thomas II, 2: 22.)*

Whenever we remember to make the two One, to resolve duality into unity, whenever we use the Unconditional Love Process, Aware Witness, Conscious Heart Focus, Balancing Breath, Holoenergetic Tracing or Forgiveness Processes to restore wholeness, we enter the Kingdom.

Any and all of these practices I have learned over a lifetime of healing with love can reconnect us to Source.

Loving Awareness

When loving awareness flows through the heart, it shifts and coheres the vibration of the inner energy-body into resonance with your essential nature — with the truth of who you really are and with the truth of what is.

Love links form with essence, the many with the One, the manifest with the unmanifest.

Loving awareness links the physical body with the inner energy-body and the energy-body with your spiritual essence. So, Love links matter with energy and energy with Spirit.

Love, at its deepest level, is the awakening to Oneness.

May we choose love, may we choose freedom, may we choose forgiveness. Now, the gates to the Kingdom are open.

FOR GIVING
LOVE

APPENDIX ONE

The Intuitive Co-Creator Process
"Freedom From" to "Freedom To"

Now that you have used the Holoenergetic Forgiveness Processes to create freedom from the past, how do you use this freedom to create a new future?

The Intuitive Co-Creator Process is a powerful tool to align your intention and will with Source so that your heart's desire can become your focused intention and therefore manifest. The Intuitive Co-Creator will help you focus the energy liberated through this process to bring more joy, peace and freedom.

Purpose: Learning to co-create your reality and manifest what you want. This can be a specific event, a state of body and mind, or even an expanded consciousness.

[Option: Start with the Grounding, Aligning, and Centering Breath and the Balancing Breath.]

RECOGNIZE

Is there something you truly want with all of your heart? If so, silently state it now. Allow yourself to sense how you would feel when it manifests. Take as much time as you need.

Where are these feelings located in your body? Do you feel it in your heart? Do you want it with all your heart in this moment? [If "yes" bypass option.]

[Option:] If not, allow yourself to sense from where the desire for this manifestation originates and what is really wanted. Reconsider what you truly want to manifest. Unless you want it with all your heart, this process will not work as efficiently.

If you truly want this with all your heart right now, silently choose and intend that this or better manifest in your life within a specific time frame.

Take whatever time you need.

Now, disengage the mind's attention — tell the mind to stop for a moment and suspend all thoughts, images, feelings, or sensations associated with this manifestation.

RESONATE

Shift attention to your heart area. Slowly and deeply breathe in and out as if through the center of your chest for at least three breaths. Allow yourself to release all effort now and just relax ... relax while breathing in and out as if through the center of your chest.

Recall a time when you felt really good, a time when you had a heart-opening experience. Focus on it and allow yourself to feel these feelings now — perhaps feelings of love, laughter, joy, inner peace, harmony, — flowing in the moment. As best you can, really feel these expansive feelings while continuing to breathe in and out through your heart center.

RELEASE

Focusing all your awareness within your heart, bring what you want into your heart. Ask your heart's intuitive wisdom, intelligence, and love to manifest your desire in the most beneficial and effective way for your highest good within the specific time frame.

When you are ready, draw a deep breath into your heart. As you release your breath, entrust your heart's desire to the universe.

REFORM

Now, allow your heart's intention to synchronistically organize the universal field of all possibilities to manifest this desired outcome.

Imagine and picture the successful outcome in your mind and feel it in your heart. Feel the gratitude in your heart in advance of the actual outcome. Feel as if it has already happened.

Finally, intend to take any action needed to bring the manifestation into being and determine the first step.

Know that manifestation has begun.

FOR GIVING
LOVE

APPENDIX TWO

The Healing Power of Love

Love is the awareness of relatedness; a relatedness to oneself, to other, and to Source.

The meaning of "relatedness" is to "carry back together." Love brings back together what was once one but seemingly became separate. It is a coming home. Love creates an energy field that affects all that enter it. It is said that the loving energy fields of Christ and Buddha were so powerful that people were healed in their presence. We might even say that the healing field of love is "magnetically resonant."

In modern medicine, there is a technique called MRI (Magnetic Resonance Imaging), which uses a magnetic field, rather than X-rays, to produce computer-generated images for diagnosis. In the blink of an eye, a magnetic field brings all the protons of the hydrogen atoms in the body into alignment, causing them all to spin and move as one. A radio wave resonant with the hydrogen proton is then pulsed through the body, producing signals that a computer translates into visual images.

MRI doesn't alter any of the protons of the other elements that constitute the body. Only the hydrogen proton flips out because only it can resonate with the pulse. When the pulse stops, the proton drops back into alignment; as it does, it releases energy. That released energy is picked up by a sensor, fed through a computer, and printed out as an image.

How is the MRI related to healing? While the energies that cause the change in MRI are generated by a magnetic field and a radio frequency resonating with the hydrogen proton, the energies that cause change in Holoenergetic Healing are generated by our love and intention. A loving field, analogous to the magnetic field in MRI, can be created by our hands, our feelings, thoughts, or our presence, especially when we are in a heightened transpersonal state.

Our intention to heal — with its attendant thoughts, feelings and images — focused by our attention, and directed by our breath can be resonantly pulsed into our body-mind, much like the radio frequency that targets the hydrogen proton in MRI. Without the magnetic field in MRI, the hydrogen proton doesn't respond to the resonant pulse — it doesn't "flip." Without the loving field in Holoenergetic Healing, the changes targeted by intention don't readily "flip" — that is, they are less likely to occur. A loving field is the activator of the body-mind, preparing it for the "healing flip," which is the resonant pulsed intention.

In the presence of a coherent magnetic field, such as that produced by MRI, the hydrogen proteins spin in concert as they align themselves with the field. In effect, they all dance the same dance; they become one. Similarly, when you create a coherent loving field, everything within that field of consciousness begins to vibrate as one to dance to the same rhythm.

When all begins to vibrate as one, separation disappears. There is only oneness. Time and space disappear because they are measures of separation. The end merges with the beginning and the spinning circle is complete. Finite becomes infinite.

In this state of oneness, the natural order and harmony inherent in the tissues, cells, molecules, atoms and subatomic particles reassert themselves. The cells remember the higher order, the balance of health and wholeness. Love is their reminder.

FOR GIVING
LOVE

APPENDIX THREE

Healer Intention

A Research Lecture Presented by Dr. Leonard Laskow.

First, I will begin with some operational definitions that I found useful in my healing work and research. Then I will present data on some of the consciousness and intention studies I have been involved with. We will look at the relative differences between thoughts and images as vehicles of intention. We will also explore the impact of love and spiritual impress on cancer cells, water, and DNA. We will see what all of this research suggests and look at some ways that we can use this information in daily living. In doing this work, I have collaborated with some gifted and creative healers who were not afraid to go to the frontiers of science, to risk the disapproval of their colleagues and to search for truth. People like Beverly Rubik and Glen Rein, Bill Tiller, Marcel Vogel, Helene and Allan Smith, and some of the folks at HeartMath. I am deeply indebted to all of them.

I would like to take a moment to share with you what inspired me to explore the role of intention in healing. It began during a retreat in the mid-seventies. It was two o'clock in the morning, I was in a deep meditation; the room was dark. Suddenly it seemed as if someone had turned on the lights. I opened my eyes and the room was still dark. Closing my eyes, I again had a sense of being filled with light. Then, I felt a presence and I heard a voice inside my head. This indescribable voice said, "Your work is to heal with love."

Tears began rolling down my cheeks, the hair stood up on the back of my head, and I silently said, "Oh so I am worthy?" This voice said, "You are no more or less worthy than anyone else. Your work is to heal with love."

See how that little ego concern came in. Worthy? This presence had nothing to do with hierarchical, egoistic considerations. I did not know at the time what this visitation meant. But as I subsequently began to work with people, I was offered synchronistic opportunities in which healing was the only option available at the moment. I was frankly surprised at the results.

I decided to explore healing with love further in the course of my Ob-Gyn practice with select patients. I had concerns that the Board of Medical Examiners would come knocking at my door one day. I was what you might call an open skeptic. The results of working with patients were remarkable and I was intrigued. I began to wonder —much as the folks at Spindrift did — How much did the placebo effect contribute to these remarkable results? How much was a manifestation of the body-mind response currently being explored by psychoneuroimmunology? How much was due to an interaction between my consciousness and that of the person whom I was working with? Because there were so many variables involved, I decided to focus my research on single-celled organisms such as bacteria and tumor cells and also on water and DNA.

I continued to work with people, but I did not do formal clinical studies. I collaborated with a friend of mine, Dr. Glen Rein, a neurobiologist who, at the time, was working at a major University in the San Francisco Bay area. We designed a series of experiments to explore the effect of different intentions generated while in non-ordinary states of consciousness. We wanted to know how these intentions would influence the growth of cancer cells in tissue culture.

I want to emphasize that these were exploratory studies designed for the purpose of discovering what was most effective. We sought to develop pilot studies that had the best chance of success. We worked under trying conditions — at night, sometimes until four or five in the morning. We worked on weekends because this research was not approved at these universities.

First, let's look at my operational definition of intention. The word "intention" is derived from Latin intenitus — a stretching toward. The American Heritage Dictionary defines intention as an aim that guides actions. Here is the definition I use: Intention is holding attention on a desired outcome with persistent and focused desire.

Attention is focused awareness that energizes the object of attention. Desire relates to the magnitude of energy associated with the intention, the feeling state. The outcome provides information that gives direction to that intention, and this information can be in the form of thought or imagery. One could say that attention aims the arrow and desired outcome draws the bow.

Another way of looking at this is in terms of energy and information. The energy of intention is provided by attention, desire and will. The information is provided by the focus on outcome, direction, goal or aim, and it can be in time and space or it can be active non-linear information which impacts distant healing. Also there are the contextual variables; the most important one is my work being the spiritual influence both consciously invoked and also superconsciously present. Then of course there are all the unconscious influences and environmental influences that make this a very complex and difficult area to study.

Now a word about the protocol. The first set of experiments involved measuring the growth of tumor cells in a culture as a biological endpoint. These were mast cell tumors that came from mouse

intestinal tissue. State of the art techniques were used to quanti-
fy the incorporation of radioactive thymidine into the DNA of the
growing cells.

I would begin the protocol by establishing what I call a "loving,
healing presence" through a transpersonal alignment and a conscious heart focus. This shifted my consciousness into a non-ordinary state. I then looked at the tumor cells that we were working
with under a microscope. I put the Petri dish containing the cells
under a microscope and came into resonance with them. I did this
by regarding them as inherently having as much right to be here as
I did even though they were cancer cells.

The energy of intention is provided by attention, desire and will.

I took a different perspective than the one most people use when
they think of cancer cells. I did the same thing when I worked with
Salmonella, bacteria that caused dysentery in humans. Coming into
resonance with them means I came into an unconditional loving acceptance of their existence as it is. When I did that, my consciousness began to vibrate at the same frequency as the cells. We became,
as it were, phase locked, perhaps entrained. Once that entrainment
took place I could then introduce intentional information and get the
most efficient result.

In other words, I learned that there was a great secret to operating on the subtle level. The secret was to focus lovingly on whatever you want to change. It seems like there is a paradox here. If
you lovingly or unconditionally accept something, why would you
change it? You are just lovingly and unconditionally accepting it.
Well, think for a moment about a child. If you unconditionally love
the child and the child does something that could be harmful to itself or to others, could you still unconditionally love the child and
yet want the child to change its behavior? Of course you could. In
fact, that may be the most loving thing to do. So there is no contradiction to healing in this particular way.

In terms of the rest of the protocol, I then held separate sets
of three Petri dishes containing these cell cultures in my hands for
each different state of consciousness or intention that we wanted to

study. In an adjacent room, a non-healer was simultaneously dupli-
cating the same protocol but was reading a book instead of focusing
on the culture cells. All the specimens were blindly labeled, scram-
bled and read after twenty-four hours. Subsequently we also treated
the water that was used to make up media without the cells to see
if water could store biological information. Then the treated and
control media were used to grow the cells.

Again, my state of consciousness was a loving acceptance, a
heart-focused resonance with the cells for all of these different contents of consciousness. The first of these three different intentions
that we studied with cells was to "Return to the natural order and
growth rate of your pre-cancer cell line." These cancer cells were
growing at an accelerated rate relative to their pre-cancerous cell
line. My interest was simply to return them to the pre-cancerous
growth rate. That was the first intention. The second intention was
to "Let God's will flow through these hands." The third intention
was simply unconditional love.

These were the results we got focusing on returning to the natural order and growth rate. There was a thirty-nine percent inhibition of the growth rate relative to the contemporaneous controls.
With "Let God's will flow through these hands," there was a twen-
ty-one percent reduction.

This is one of the challenges in doing work with subtle information and subtle energy in healing.

Interestingly, with unconditional love, there was no change. But
if you stop to think about it, when you unconditionally love something and you totally accept it as it is, from the perspective of the
consciousness of these tumor cells, they say, "Great, we will continue to do our thing." We did not give them any direction via intention. The direction associated with unconditional love can come
from conscious or superconscious or unconscious forces. I did the
best I could to simply unconditionally love them without intentions.

As I mentioned, we also focused on the water that was used to
make up media to grow these cells. Again we used three different
intentions: "Return to the natural order," "unconditional love" and

"dematerialize into the light." (I was interested in exploring the differences between dematerializing into the light or into the void to see if a cell's consciousness would have a preference between the two. I wondered whether single celled organisms had a fear of "dematerializing into the void," much as people have. However, in this series we used "dematerialize into the light."

"Return to the natural order" resulted in a twenty-nine percent inhabitation of growth rate relative to contemporaneous controls. This time, with "unconditional love" there was a twenty-two percent inhibition of growth rate and "dematerialize into the light" produced a twenty-nine percent inhibition. But I had a consideration when I went over the results because I had charged three flasks of water and we stored these flasks next to one another for three months before we used this water to make up the media for these experiments. There was good news and there was bad news from this experiment. The good news is that water stores biologically active information for at least three months. The bad news was that there may have been a resonant transfer of information from one flask to another since there was an unexpected effect from the unconditional love.

When I give seminars, I have people charge wine and water as a group after establishing transpersonal alignment and conscious heart focus. We can actually smell and taste the difference between the charged wine and uncharged wine, the charged water and uncharged water. If you leave the two in relative proximity to one another over a period of time, there is less and less difference. On the other hand, if you separate them at least five feet, then over time there is a greater difference between charged and the uncharged liquid.

My concern was that there is some exchange of information and perhaps energy when they are in proximity. This is one of the challenges in doing work with subtle information and subtle energy in healing. Also, if you do not clear your intention after each set, the next intent can be contaminated by the previous intent. It is that subtle.

Next, I was interested in exploring the relative impact of thought vs. imagery on the growth of cancer cells. This time I used different initiating intents. Again, the first intention was "Return to the natural order and growth rate of your pre-cancerous cell line" which produced and eighteen percent inhibition of cell growth. Then, as I held the thought of returning to the natural order, I also introduced an image. Since the Petri dishes that we worked with contained quite a few cells covering almost the entire surface of the media, I imagined just three cells in the culture. When I did that the result was a thirty-nine percent inhibition, implying that adding imagery to thought doubles the effectiveness of intention.

The next time instead of holding natural order as an initial intent, I simply circulated energy. Now all of this, of course, was still done while in loving resonance with the cells, using the same protocol as before. So there was an overall loving field in which this was taking place.

In circulating energy, I sensed and imagined my attention moving up my spine and down the front of my body. I would breathe in through the Hara or Dan Tien about two finger breadths below my navel, down to the base of my spine, up my spine, and through the crown and around the transpersonal space above my head and down the front of my body and back into the Hara. When I did that, I did not hold a thought of "returning to the natural order" but did hold the image of just three cells, and in that situation we got an eighteen percent inhibition of cell growth. Then I repeated the experiment circulating energy again but this time holding the image of many cells, and we got a fifteen percent increase. In other words, we were able to reverse the intention and stimulate growth by fifteen percent. In summary then, when we add thought to imagery or imagery to thought, we can double the impact of our healing intention. And also we can reverse it.

Eventually we lost our lab access, so we started looking for a different experimental end point. We decided to explore modulating the molecular confirmation of DNA by winding it or unwinding it. We worked with human placental DNA dissolved in water that had distinctive characteristic patterns when measured with ultraviolet spectroscopy.

I would enter into this loving state and have the intention of un-winding the double helix of DNA using both thought and imagery. Folks at an organization called the Institute of HeartMath heard what we were doing and invited me to come by. They monitored me with an electrocardiogram, electroencephalogram, and electromy-elogram, ran the leads to a computer to process the data. We found when I was in these non-ordinary states of consciousness and was able to unwind the double helixes of DNA, the frequency power spectrum revealed a state of internal coherence. I could also inten-tionally rewind DNA that had been heated or denatured, in effect bringing the two DNA strands together again. In order for DNA to replicate, it needs to unwind, so there are implications here for our biology.

When we add thought to imagery or imagery to thought we can double the impact of our healing intention.

And also we can reverse it.

When we looked at the frequency power spectrum of someone who was not trained in these methods but who was trying to love, there was a lack of coherence. Coherence is what makes laser light so powerful. As energy is cohered it is squared. When you come into cardiac coherence, the energy is squared and whatever you focus your attention upon becomes dramatically amplified and has greater impact. You become laser-like.

At the Institute of HeartMath, ten people who were trained in these methods of heart coherence were asked to focus their inten-tion on DNA, and they were able to unwind it. Ten others who were not trained in these methods were asked to hold the same intention, but were unable to unwind the DNA.

In another experiment I was interested in finding out what would happen if, instead of my intention, I called upon spiritual impress to influence the molecular confirmation of DNA. I silently said, "I ask that you manifest your spiritual presence on the material plane in such way that science can acknowledge it. I will not take personal credit for the results." What I heard was, "We know what you say is true. Just remain with your eyes closed, relax and be still." Then I felt a shift that I can only describe as an expansive emptiness having fullness to it. That worked to unwind the DNA and then when we heated the DNA and repeated the experiment the denatured DNA was rewound. So this demonstrated that we are able to work with spirit in a way that really manifests its presence.

I want to close with a word of caution about extrapolating these results to human beings because people have their own countervailing intentions both conscious and unconscious. That has a tremendous impact on the healing response. Also I would just like to simply remind you of what you already know. We are all graced with spirit, which flows through us, and this flow can be enhanced as we lovingly ask and allow it to be. Then the creative separation of individuation becomes the conscious recognition of unity.

Published in the Fall, 1999 issue of Bridges, ISSSEEM Magazine, Volume 10, Number 3

FOR GIVING
LOVE

ABOUT THE AUTHOR

LEONARD LASKOW Is a Stanford-trained Life Fellow of the American College of Obstetrics and Gynecology, former Chief of OB-GYN at the Community Hospital of the Monterey Peninsula in Carmel, California, and has served as faculty at the University of California, San Francisco. He was a founding diplomate of the American Board of Integrative Holistic Medicine and a former member of HeartMath Institute's Scientific Advisory Board. He served as a US Naval Flight Surgeon in Vietnam.

Dr. Laskow has done seminal research with biophysicists, neuro-chemists, and crystallographers on the impact of information and coherent energy on cancer cells, DNA, the growth of bacteria, and water. His acclaimed book, Healing with Love has been published in nine languages. Currently, he resides in Switzerland and is a consultant in Behavioral Medicine lecturing and giving seminars internationally. His website is www.laskow.net and he has received the Worldwide Forgiveness Alliance's Champion of Forgiveness Award

In collaboration with

STEVE BHAERMAN is an author and humorist who's spent the past twenty-eight years writing and performing comedy as Swami Beyondananda. Author Marianne Williamson calls him "The Mark Twain of our generation." On the serious side, Steve is the author of Spontaneous Evolution: Our Positive Future and a Way to Get There from Here, written with Bruce Lipton. Since 2006, he has written a political / spiritual blog called Notes from the Trail bringing humor and perspective to challenging times. His website is www.wakeuplaughing.com.

Made in the USA
San Bernardino, CA
23 December 2016